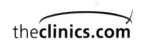

ORTHOPEDIC CLINICS
OF NORTH AMERICA

Shoulder Trauma

GUEST EDITOR
George S. Athwal, MD, FRCSC

October 2008 • Volume 39 • Number 4

SAUNDERS

An Imprint of Elsevier, Inc.
PHILADELPHIA   LONDON   TORONTO   MONTREAL   SYDNEY   TOKYO

W.B. SAUNDERS COMPANY
A Division of Elsevier Inc.

Elsevier Inc., 1600 John F. Kennedy Blvd., Suite 1800, Philadelphia, PA 19103-2899.

http://www.orthopedic.theclinics.com

ORTHOPEDIC CLINICS OF NORTH AMERICA   Volume 39, Number 4
October 2008   ISSN 0030-5898
Editor: Debora Dellapena   ISBN-10: 1-4160-6331-5
          ISBN-13: 978-1-4160-6331-5

Orthopedic Clinics of North America (ISSN 0030-5898) is published quarterly (For Post Office use only: Volume 39 issue 4 of 4) by Elsevier Inc., 360 Park Avenue South, New York, NY 10010-1710. Months of publication are January, April, July, and October. Business and Editorial Offices: 1600 John F. Kennedy Blvd., Suite 1800, Philadelphia, PA 19103-2899. Customer Service Office: 6277 Sea Harbor Drive, Orlando, FL 33887-4800. Periodicals postage paid at New York, NY and additional mailing offices. Subscription prices are $244.00 per year for (US individuals), $424.00 per year for (US institutions), $288.00 per year (Canadian individuals), $508.00 per year (Canadian institutions), $355.00 per year (international individuals), $508.00 per year (international institutions), $122.00 per year (US students), $177.00 per year (Canadian and international students). Foreign air speed delivery is included in all *Clinics* subscription prices. All prices are subject to change without notice. **POSTMASTER:** Send address changes to *Orthopedic Clinics of North America*, Elsevier Periodicals Customer Service, 6277 Sea Harbor Drive, Orlando, FL 32887-4800. **Customer Service: 1-800-654-2452 (US). From outside the United States, call 1-407-563-6020. Fax: 1-407-363-9661. E-mail: JournalsCustomerService-usa@elsevier.com.**

Reprints. For copies of 100 or more of articles in this publication, please contact the Commercial Reprints Department, Elsevier Inc., 360 Park Avenue South, New York, NY 10010-1710. Tel.: 212-633-3812; Fax: 212-462-1935; E-mail: reprints@elsevier.com.

Orthopedic Clinics of North America is covered in *MEDLINE/PubMed* (*Index Medicus*), *Cinahl, Excerpta Medica, and Cumulative Index to Nursing and Allied Health Literature.*

Printed in the United States of America.

GUEST EDITOR

GEORGE S. ATHWAL, MD, FRCSC, Consultant and Assistant Professor of Surgery, Hand and Upper Limb Centre, St Joseph's Health Care, University of Western Ontario, London, Ontario, Canada

CONTRIBUTORS

GEORGE S. ATHWAL, MD, FRCSC, Consultant and Assistant Professor of Surgery, Hand and Upper Limb Centre, St Joseph's Health Care, University of Western Ontario, London, Ontario, Canada

PHILLIP W. BENNION, MD, Shoulder and Elbow Service, The Carrell Clinic, Dallas, Texas

WAYNE Z. BURKHEAD, MD, Shoulder and Elbow Service, The Carrell Clinic, Dallas, Texas

EMILIE V. CHEUNG, MD, Assistant Professor, Department of Orthopedic Surgery, Stanford University, Stanford, California

FRANK A. CORDASCO, MD, Attending Surgeon, Sports Medicine and Shoulder Service, Hospital for Special Surgery; Associate Professor of Orthopaedic Surgery, Cornell University, Weill Medical College, New York, New York

CHRISTOPHER C. DODSON, MD, Fellow, Sports Medicine and Shoulder Service, Hospital for Special Surgery, New York, New York

DARREN S. DROSDOWECH, MD, FRCSC, Hand and Upper Limb Centre, St. Joseph's Health Care; Department of Surgery, University of Western Ontario, London, Ontario, Canada

KENNETH J. FABER, MD, MHPE, FRCSC, Hand and Upper Limb Centre, St. Joseph's Health Care; Department of Surgery, University of Western Ontario, London, Ontario, Canada

JEFFERY S. HUGHES, MBBS, FRACS, FAOrthA, Sydney Shoulder and Elbow Associates, Sydney, New South Wales, Australia

JOSEPH P. IANNOTTI, MD, PhD, Maynard Madden Professor and Chairman, Orthopaedic and Rheumatologic Institute, Department of Orthopaedic Surgery, Cleveland Clinic, Cleveland Clinic Lerner College of Medicine, Cleveland, Ohio

WON KIM, MD, Resident, Division of Orthopaedic Surgery, St. Michaels Hospital and the University of Toronto, Toronto, Ontario, Canada

MARC S. KOWALSKY, MD, Chief Resident, Department of Orthopaedic Surgery, Center for Shoulder, Elbow, and Sports Medicine, Columbia University Medical Center, New York, New York

SUMANT G. KRISHNAN, MD, Shoulder and Elbow Service, The Carrell Clinic, Dallas, Texas

PETER C. LAPNER, MD, FRCSC, Assistant Professor, Division of Orthopedics, University of Ottawa, The Ottawa Hospital, Ottawa, Ontario, Canada

PIERRE LAPOINTE, MD, FRCSC, Fellow in Orthopaedic Sport Medicine and Upper Extremity Reconstruction, Pan Am Clinic, University of Manitoba, Manitoba, Canada

WILLIAM N. LEVINE, MD, Vice Chairman and Professor, Department of Orthopaedic Surgery, Center for Shoulder, Elbow, and Sports Medicine, Columbia University Medical Center, New York, New York

PETER B. MACDONALD, MD, FRCSC, Professor and Head; Gibson Chair of Orthopaedic Surgery and Research, Section of Orthopaedic Surgery, University of Manitoba, Manitoba, Canada

BRIAN MAGOVERN, MD, Fellow, Shoulder and Elbow Service, Department of Orthopaedic Surgery, Thomas Jefferson University, Philadelphia, Pennsylvania

THOMAS G. MARTIN, BS, Medical Student, Case Western Reserve University, School of Medicine, Cleveland, Ohio

MICHAEL D. McKEE, MD, FRCS(C), Professor of Surgery, Division of Orthopaedic Surgery, St. Michael's Hospital and the University of Toronto, Toronto, Ontario, Canada

STEVE PAPP, MD, FRCSC, Assistant Professor, Division of Orthopedics, University of Ottawa, The Ottawa Hospital, Ottawa, Ontario, Canada

MATTHEW L. RAMSEY, MD, Associate Professor of Orthopaedic Surgery, Rothman Institute, Thomas Jefferson University, Philadelphia, Pennsylvania

JOHN R. REINECK, MD, Shoulder and Elbow Service, The Carrell Clinic, Dallas, Texas

DAMIAN M. RISPOLI, MD, Department Chairman and Chief of Shoulder and Elbow Surgery, Department of Orthopaedics, Wilford Hall Medical Center, Lackland Air Force Base, Texas; Assistant Professor of Surgery, F. Edward Hebert School of Medicine, Uniformed Services University, Bethesda, Maryland

BEN C. ROBINSON, MD, Orthopaedic Surgery Resident, Department of Orthopaedics, Wilford Hall Medical Center, Lackland Air Force Base, Texas

JOAQUIN SANCHEZ-SOTELO, MD, PhD, Consultant and Associate Professor of Orthopedics, Mayo Clinic, Rochester, Minnesota

JOHN W. SPERLING, MD, Associate Professor, Department of Orthopedic Surgery, Mayo Clinic, Rochester, Minnesota

SCOTT P. STEINMANN, MD, Mayo Clinic, Department of Orthopaedic Surgery, Rochester, Minnesota

THOMAS W. THROCKMORTON, MD, Mayo Clinic, Department of Orthopaedic Surgery, Rochester, Minnesota

HANS K. UHTHOFF, MD, FRCSC, Professor Emeritus, Division of Orthopedics, University of Ottawa, The Ottawa Hospital, Ottawa, Ontario, Canada

ALLAN A. YOUNG, MBBS, MSpMed, PhD, Department of Orthopaedic and Traumatic Surgery, Royal North Shore Hospital, Sydney, NSW, Australia

PETER C. ZARKADAS, MD, FRCS(C), Mayo Clinic, Department of Orthopaedic Surgery, Rochester, Minnesota

CONTRIBUTORS

CONTENTS

approach with limited soft tissue dissection, achieve accurate anatomic reduction, provide a secure construct even in the situation of osteopenic bone or comminution, and manage fractures of the proximal humerus extending into the shaft.

Open Reduction and Internal Fixation of Proximal Humerus Fractures 429
Darren S. Drosdowech, Kenneth J. Faber, and George S. Athwal

Open reduction of proximal humeral fractures has the advantage of providing direct control over each fracture fragment and permitting anatomic reduction and fixation with advanced devices. Modern fixed-angle locking plates designed specifically for proximal humerus fractures have allowed the expansion of surgical indications permitting surgeons to address more complicated fractures. Advanced preoperative imaging and fluoroscopy allow a better understanding of fracture patterns and permit the surgeon to use this knowledge intraoperatively. Research is required to further validate fracture classification systems, to develop surgical guidelines for decision making, and to compare the outcomes of the various treatments options for proximal humerus fractures.

Hemiarthroplasty for Proximal Humeral Fracture: Restoration of the Gothic Arch 441
Sumant G. Krishnan, Phillip W. Bennion, John R. Reineck, and Wayne Z. Burkhead

Proximal humerus fractures are the most common fractures of the shoulder girdle, and initial management of these injuries often determines final outcome. When arthroplasty is used to manage proximal humeral fractures, surgery remains technically demanding, and outcomes have been unpredictable. Recent advances in both technique and prosthetic implants have led to more successful and reproducible results. Key technical points include restoration of the Gothic arch, anatomic tuberosity reconstruction, and minimal soft tissue dissection.

Reverse Total Shoulder Arthroplasty for Acute Fractures and Failed Management After Proximal Humeral Fractures 451
Thomas G. Martin and Joseph P. Iannotti

Reverse shoulder arthroplasty (RSA) has a successful clinical record when used for treatment of arthropathy accompanied by rotator cuff insufficiency. Efforts to use the same technology for other conditions involving insufficient cuff function are related to proximal humeral fracture described in this review for which RSA has shown promise are treatment of failed hemiarthroplasty for treatment of proximal humeral fractures and treatment of complex fracture sequelae. Specific conclusions as yet are difficult to reach. Future studies are needed to determine if supplemental soft tissue procedures or modification of implant design will serve to improve functional outcome in this difficult-to-treat subset of patients.

Scapula Fractures 459
Peter C. Lapner, Hans K. Uhthoff, and Steve Papp

Fractures of the scapula are rare and the diagnosis and treatment may be unfamiliar to some surgeons. This article outlines a diagnostic work-up and treatment approach for the various types of scapular fractures. The approach helps guide decision making on operative versus nonoperative treatment based on what is known regarding prognosis and outcomes of management. Operative technique and fixation strategies are discussed for the common fracture patterns along with guidelines for postsurgical shoulder rehabilitation.

FORTHCOMING ISSUES

RECENT ISSUES

ORTHOPEDIC
CLINICS
OF NORTH AMERICA

Orthop Clin N Am 39 (2008) xi–xii

Preface

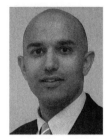

George S. Athwal, MD, FRCSC
Guest Editor

The past decade has brought significant change to the understanding, evaluation, and treatment of shoulder trauma. This issue of *Orthopedic Clinics of North America* is dedicated to shoulder trauma and discusses these current developments, providing guidance on their clinical and technical applications. This issue is made possible through the efforts of its contributing authors—a nationally and internationally renowned group.

The first article by Dr. Robinson and colleagues outlines the basics of imaging and describes the many classification systems specific to fractures of the proximal humerus. Recognizing that there are several controversies in the management of proximal humerus fractures and that there may be many "correct" treatment methods, the authors of the next four articles were charged with defending their preferred techniques (see the articles by Drs. Hughes and Young; Drs. Magovern and Ramsey; Dr. Drosdowech and colleagues; and Dr. Krishnan and colleagues).

The article by Drs. Martin and Iannotti eloquently describes the expanding roles of reverse total shoulder arthroplasty with specific attention to acute fractures and revision procedures. Dr. Lapner's article provides an excellent overview of scapular and glenoid fractures.

Drs. Cheung and Sperling and Dr. Zarkadas and coauthors share their experiences with the management of associated injures and complications of shoulder trauma. The review by Drs. Kim and McKee addresses the controversies surrounding clavicle fractures, with special attention to the changing role of surgery. The articles by Drs. Dodson and Cordasco and Drs. Kowalsky and Levine provide an excellent overview and approach to the management of complex shoulder instability. Finally, the discussion by Dr. MacDonald and colleagues outlines the management of acromioclavicular and sternoclavicular joint trauma.

It is an exciting time for shoulder trauma with the advent of advanced imaging, precontoured locking plates, fracture-specific prosthesis, and reverse shoulder arthroplasty. Just as important, the development of disease-specific, patient-specific, and limb-specific outcome measures will objectively determine the value of these advances.

This issue would not have been possible without the outstanding skill and support of Debora Dellapena, Acquisitions Editor of *Orthopedic Clinics of North America*. She engineered a painstakingly precise schedule, and then enforced it. I would also like to thank my mentors at Queen's University, the Hospital for

orthopedic.theclinics.com

Special Surgery, the Mayo Clinic, and the University of Western Ontario for their support and guidance.

I would like to thank and dedicate this issue to my wife Lorraine and my son Marcus.

George S. Athwal, MD, FRCSC
Hand and Upper Limb Centre
St Joseph's Health Care
University of Western Ontario
268 Grosvenor Street
London, Ontario, Canada, N6A 4L6

E-mail address: gathwal@uwo.ca

ELSEVIER
SAUNDERS

Orthop Clin N Am 39 (2008) 393–403

ORTHOPEDIC
CLINICS
OF NORTH AMERICA

Classification and Imaging of Proximal Humerus Fractures

Ben C. Robinson, MD[a], George S. Athwal, MD, FRCSC[b],
Joaquin Sanchez-Sotelo, MD, PhD[c],
Damian M. Rispoli, MD[a,d],*

[a]Department of Orthopaedics, Wilford Hall Medical Center, 2200 Bergquist Drive,
Suite 1, Lackland AFB, TX 78236, USA
[b]Hand and Upper Limb Centre, St Joesph's Health Care, University of Western Ontario, 268 Grosvenor Street,
London, Ontario, Canada, N6A 4L6
[c]Mayo Clinic, 200 First Street SW, Rochester, MN 55905, USA
[d]F. Edward Hebert School of Medicine, Uniformed Services University, Bethesda, MD 20814, USA

Fractures of the proximal humerus represent the second most common fracture type of the upper extremity and the third most common fracture in patients older than 65 years after hip and distal radius fractures [1]. In the past, surgical treatment has been estimated to be required in 20% of proximal humerus fractures. The indications for surgery continue to expand for several reasons, including a better understanding of the multiple fracture patterns, higher patient expectations, and improvements in internal fixation techniques, hemiarthroplasty, tuberosity reconstruction, and the selective use of modern reverse prosthesis designs.

The decision to operate and the selection of the appropriate surgical modality for proximal humerus fractures are largely based on the fracture pattern. Understanding the particular fracture pattern in each case is complicated, however, especially when poorly positioned radiographs are the only available studies. Most well-accepted classification systems were developed based on radiographs complemented by intraoperative findings. Three-dimensional reconstructions based on

CT currently available in most institutions allow a much better understanding of complex fractures.

The ultimate goal of any classification scheme is to allow for determination of the best treatment of each individual fracture, and subsequently the ability to compare efficacy of various treatment methods on a particular fracture. The most influential early innovative concepts related to the understanding of proximal humerus fractures were introduced by Codman in 1934. Codman [2] classified proximal humeral fractures as occurring between the humeral head, shaft, and lesser or greater tuberosity (Fig. 1). Neer [3] was responsible for the second major advancement in proximal humerus fracture understanding by developing the concepts of Codman and proposing a classification system based on fracture pathoanatomy. Emphasis on the vascularity of the proximal humerus led to a deeper understanding of fracture configuration as related to perfusion of the articular segment. The AO (Arbeitsgemeinschaft für Osteosynthesefragen) classification highlights vascularity in their classification system. Most existing classification systems focus on the anatomy of the fracture fragments [3] or the anatomy of the fracture fragments with a secondary focus on vascular anatomy [4]. Some classifications use newer imaging modalities [5], such as CT, which has led to a greater level of information being available for decision making in the treatment of these fractures.

* Corresponding author. Department of Orthopaedics, Wilford Hall Medical Center, Lackland AFB, 2200 Bergquist Drive, Suite 1, TX 78236.

E-mail address: damian.rispoli@lackland.af.mil (D.M. Rispoli).

0030-5898/08/$ - see front matter. Published by Elsevier Inc.
doi:10.1016/j.ocl.2008.05.002

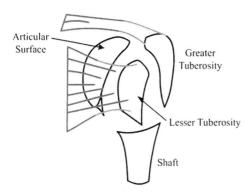

Fig. 1. Four segments of proximal humeral fractures. (*Courtesy of* D. M. Rispoli, MD, Lackland AFB, TX.)

Classification systems

Neer classification

In 1970, Neer [3] published his classification of proximal humerus fractures. Traditional classification schemes focused on the mechanism of injury [6,7] or on the level of the fracture [8,9]. Neer noted that fracture level was of little assistance, as proximal humeral fractures frequently involved multiple levels. Additionally, these classification systems placed displaced and nondisplaced fractures in similar categories. Neer based his pathoanatomic classification system (Fig. 2) on the study of the radiographic and intraoperative anatomy of 300 displaced proximal humeral fractures and fracture-dislocations treated at his institution by closed reduction under anesthesia or surgery. His system is based on the presence or absence of displacement of one or more of the four major bony segments: the surgical neck, the anatomic neck, the greater tuberosity, and the lesser tuberosity. By dividing the fractures in this manner the surgeon could focus on the deforming forces of the muscular attachments, the circulatory status of the fragments, and the continuity of the articular surface.

Displacement was defined as more than 1 cm of separation or more than 45 degrees of angulation between fragments. The decision to define displacement by this criterion was based on an editorial suggestion and has been noted by Neer [10] to have been "arbitrarily set." He further clarified that it was not intended to dictate treatment but simply to define the minimal displacement category (one part), aid in decision making, and aid in standardization of future outcome studies [10]. The reference points for measurements of displacement and angulation

between the different fragments have never been clearly defined.

The six subgroups of the original classification, designated by Roman numerals I through VI, were changed in 1975. Neer [10] stated in his 2002 paper in the *Journal of Shoulder and Elbow Surgery* that, "the 4-segment classification is not meant to be a numerical classification that is oversimplified or patterned for easy roentgen classification, but rather is a 'concept' or mental picture of the actual pathomechanics and pathoanatomy of displaced humeral fractures and the terminology to identify each category." In the original study, radiographic assessment was performed using an anteroposterior radiograph perpendicular to the scapular plane and a scapular Y view [3]. Subsequently, a three-view series was recommended, including an axillary view [11,12]. Neer's system of classification has been widely used for close to 40 years and much has been published in the literature regarding it, including its reliability and efficacy.

AO classification

The AO classification system is also widely used and accepted for fracture classification of the proximal humerus, especially in Europe (Fig. 3). This system was based on a study of 730 cases and classifies fractures into A, B, or C types, depending on whether the fractures are (A) extra-articular, unifocal, with intact vascular supply; (B) extra-articular, bifocal, with possible vascular compromise; or (C) articular, with a high likelihood of vascular compromise. Each type is then further divided into groups and then subgroups depending on fracture location, impaction, displacement, dislocation, angulation, or malalignment, resulting in multiple different possibilities [13].

In 1996, the Orthopaedic Trauma Association adopted the original AO system developed by Marsh and colleagues [4] with the goal of classifying fractures in a "uniform and consistent" manner allowing for "standardization of research and communication." This system was again modified in 2007 in the hopes of further stimulating interest in a unified fracture classification language resulting in improved patient care and clinical research. The advantages of a comprehensive system include providing a universal language for fracture communication whereby clear definitions exist for various fracture types. Recognized difficulties of this system are its complexity and observer disagreement [4].

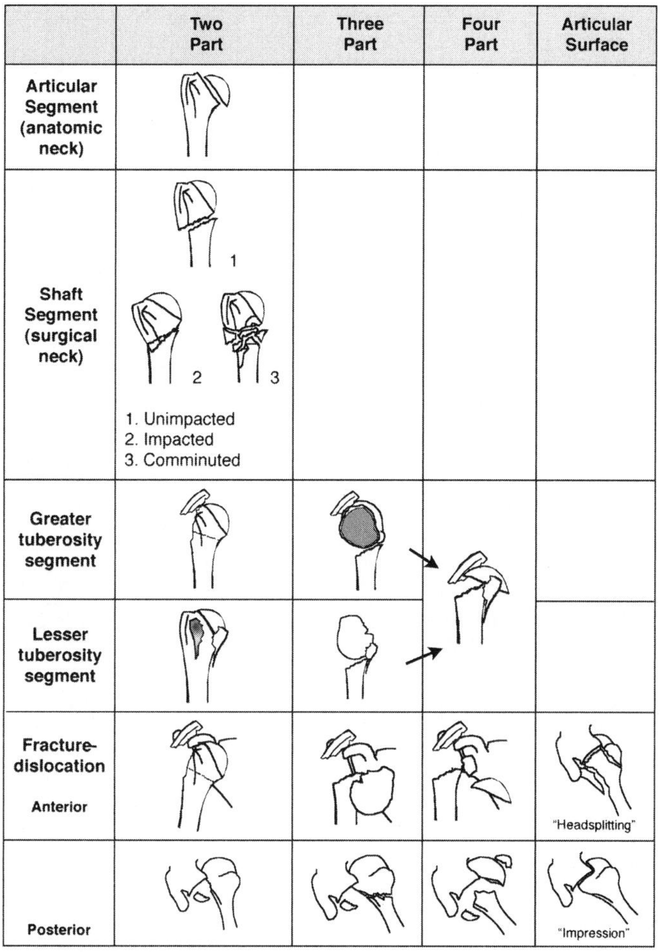

	Two Part	Three Part	Four Part	Articular Surface
Articular Segment (anatomic neck)				
Shaft Segment (surgical neck)	1 2 3 1. Unimpacted 2. Impacted 3. Comminuted			
Greater tuberosity segment				
Lesser tuberosity segment				
Fracture-dislocation Anterior				"Headsplitting"
Posterior				"Impression"

Fig. 2. The Neer classification of proximal humeral fractures. (*Adapted from* Neer CS. Four-segment classification of proximal humeral fractures: purpose and reliable use. J Shoulder Elbow Surg 2002;11(4):391; with permission.)

Edelson CT classification system

Edelson and colleagues [5] described a three-dimensional (3-D) classification system of proximal humerus fractures. The authors studied 73 museum specimens selected from more than 3200 specimens examined and 84 3-D CT reconstructions from their own clinical cases. The examined specimens were complicated fracture patterns correlating to Neer three- or four-part fractures. Five major fracture patterns were identified: two-part, three-part, "shield" fractures and their variants, isolated greater tuberosity, and fracture-dislocations.

The authors attributed most fractures of the proximal humerus to the position in which the arm was held when trying to break a fall, namely forward flexion, abduction, and internal rotation.

The authors describe the glenoid like an anvil on which the proximal humerus fractures. Other recognized mechanisms of injury were a direct impact to the proximal humerus or a fall with the arm in external rotation.

Two-part fractures most often consisted of the head with the tuberosities attached and a fracture through the weaker metaphyseal bone of the surgical neck. Three-part fractures were the most common multipart fracture. They consisted of the head with the lesser tuberosity, the greater tuberosity, and a surgical neck fracture. The superior portion of the bicipital groove remained intact in this fracture pattern; therefore, the authors suggested there was preservation of the major blood supply to the humeral head by way of the anterior circumflex vessels.

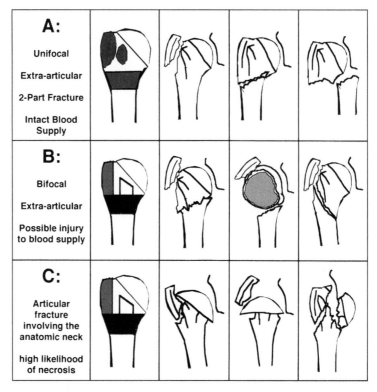

Fig. 3. The AO classification of proximal humeral fractures. (*Data from* Marsh JL, Slongo T, Agel J, et al. Fracture and dislocation classification compendium—2007. J Orthop Trauma 2007;21(Suppl 10):S1–133.)

The shield fracture was a progression of the three-part fracture and occurred when the head segment was further driven down and back. The shield was defined as the section of bone circling the head composed of the greater and lesser tuberosities and held together by the bicipital groove. The shield fracture pattern involved the superior bicipital groove and the lesser tuberosity, with the shield fragment itself usually being comminuted. Isolated fractures of the greater tuberosity were more commonly on the posterolateral aspect of the greater tuberosity and did not extend into the bicipital groove.

The final category was fracture-dislocations, with anterior dislocation mechanisms occurring with external rotation and posterior dislocations with internal rotation. The fracture component mirrored the patterns seen in fractures without associated dislocations.

Evaluation of current classification systems

Evaluation of the classification systems for fractures of the proximal humerus with plain radiographs has yielded low interobserver reliability [14–20]. In an attempt to increase reliability CT has been added as an adjunct to radiographs with varied results [14,17,21–24]. Castagno and colleagues [21] and Guix and colleagues [24] found CT beneficial; Bernstein and colleagues [14] and Sjödén and colleagues [23] noted no additional benefit. Even the inclusion of 3-D CT imaging did not improve reliability [17,22]. The experience of the surgeon has been shown to improve reliability in two studies [12,22] and not to alter reliability in one [17]. Reduction of the classification complexity has not been shown to improve reliability [12,14], whereas formal training and a structured protocol have been shown to improve reliability [15,24]. Siebenrock and Gerber [19] evaluated the Neer and AO/American Society for Internal Fixation systems showing similar concerns for both systems.

Using the 3-D classification system, interobserver reproducibility was 0.69. The authors concluded that using a 3-D versus a two-dimensional system of classification to guide treatment options was significantly better and it had the potential to "modify and improve surgical procedures" [5] to include less destructive approaches and more anatomic reconstruction. Limitations of the classification system were secondary to limitations of 3-D technology, especially in recreating fractures that were minimally displaced or severely comminuted, and lack of rapid reconstruction and ease of acquisition. The CT classification has not gained widespread use.

Many concerns regarding the current classification systems have been expressed in the literature. None have evaluated Dr. Neer's classification system in the manner it was designed (ie, using operative findings correlated with radiographs to arrive at the final classification) [10]. The Neer classification system has received support from surgeons by its use in clinical studies, practice, and the orthopaedic literature [25].

Imaging studies

Bone density assessment

Critical evaluation of the radiographic and clinical parameters to determine physiologic age is more appropriate than decisions based on chronologic age. One part of the decision-making process on the treatment of proximal humerus fractures is based on bone quality—specifically the presence or absence of osteoporosis. Bone mineral density can be roughly determined by radiographic evaluation and can have a considerable effect on treatment options [26]. Tingart and colleagues [27] identified a reliable and reproducible predictor of bone mineral density of the proximal humerus. They compared the cortical thickness of the proximal humeral diaphysis with the bone mineral density of the proximal humerus. They noted that a cortical thickness (defined as the sum of the cortical thickness of the medial and lateral cortex of the proximal humerus) less than 4 mm was highly predictive of low bone mineral density (Fig. 4). The critical evaluation of plain radiographs has been reported as a better predictor of osteopenia than simple age-based criteria [28]. Additionally the radiographic images must be evaluated for the presence of an intact medial buttress because this has been theorized to be important in strength of fixation, especially regarding current locking plate technology [29].

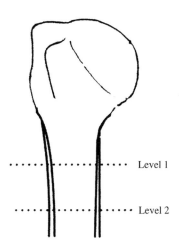

Level 1: The most proximal aspect of the humeral diaphysis in which the endosteal borders of the medial and lateral cortices are parallel
Level 2: 20 mm distal to Level 1

Level 1 + 2 > 4 mm
needed for adequate screw purchase

Fig. 4. Combined cortical thickness. (*From* Tingart MJ, Apreleva M, von Stechow D, et al. The cortical thickness of the proximal humerus diaphysis predicts bone mineral density of the proximal jumerus. J Bone Joint Surg Br 2003;85:611–7; with permission.)

Radiographic evaluation of vascularity

Another consideration in the radiographic classification of proximal humeral fractures is the vascularity of the humeral head. Avascular necrosis is a known sequelae of proximal humeral fractures and has been reported at rates of 21% to 75% [30,31]. Fracture nonunion and tuberosity reabsorption may also be influenced by fracture vascularity. The vascularity of the humeral head segment in conjunction with the state of the articular surface and other mitigating patient factors help to determine optimum treatment. The vascularity of the proximal humerus has been well studied by different groups (Fig. 5) [32–36]. The vascular supply of the humeral head is presumed damaged in four-part fractures unless the medial aspect of the fracture line lies below the articular surface, preserving some of the medial capsular vessels. Hertel and colleagues [37] devised a series of criteria that could be predictive of humeral head ischemia after fracture (Fig. 6). They viewed the tuberosities as intercalated segments between

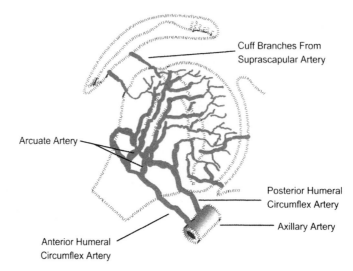

Cuff Branches From
Suprascapular Artery

Arcuate Artery

Posterior Humeral
Circumflex Artery

Axillary Artery

Anterior Humeral
Circumflex Artery

Fig. 5. The vascularity of the proximal humerus. (*Courtesy of* D. M. Rispoli, MD, Lackland AFB, TX.)

the head and the shaft instead of the classic view in which the tuberosities were protuberances of the metaphysis. Specific fracture combinations were associated with impaired head perfusion. Fractures that were predictive of ischemia were those of the anatomic neck, four-part displaced, and all three-part fractures configurations except one. The exception three-part fracture that maintained perfusion involved a fracture at the anatomic neck and a fracture below the tuberosities at the surgical neck; however, the tuberosities did not have a fracture between them. Additional elements, such as length of the posteromedial metaphyseal extension (<8 mm associated with vascular compromise) and the integrity of the medial hinge, were also key in predicting vascular disruption. They noted that the degree of displacement of the four components was less important

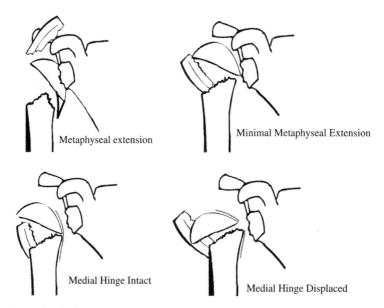

Metaphyseal extension

Minimal Metaphyseal Extension

Medial Hinge Intact

Medial Hinge Displaced

Fig. 6. Hertel radiographic criteria. (*Redrawn from* Hertal R, Hempfing A, Stiehler M, et al. Predictors of humeral head ischemia after intracapsular fracture of the proximal humerus. J Shoulder Elbow Surg 2004;13:429; with permission.)

than the key elements they noted. Certain displaced fractures, notably the valgus impacted fractures, have been theorized to cause less destruction of the proximal humeral blood supply theoretically because of preservation of the medial hinge and subsequently the posteromedial vasculature [38].

Tamai and colleagues [39] suggested that the orientation of the articular surface is important in predicting humeral head vascularity. The absence of displacement or medial displacement of the humeral head with respect to the humeral shaft was predictive of maintained vascularity to the humeral head.

Radiographs

In his landmark publication, Neer [3] suggested that determination of fracture configuration could be done using true anteroposterior (AP) and scapular Y radiographs. Over the years, others suggested the need for an additional radiographic view, the axillary lateral [11,12,14,15, 40–42]. The axillary radiograph best shows displacement of the lesser and greater tuberosities and splits and dislocations of the humeral head.

A trauma series of radiographs represents the minimum requirement in the evaluation of proximal humerus fractures. This series consists of a true anteroposterior view of the scapula and glenohumeral joint, an axillary view, and a lateral Y view of the scapula. The trauma series evaluates the glenohumeral joint and proximal humerus in three perpendicular planes.

The true AP view is shot with the beam angled 45 degrees from the sagittal plane (perpendicular to the axis of the scapula). This view projects clearly the articular surface of the humeral head and the joint space from the glenoid fossa. This view is also a good image for evaluation of the tuberosities (Fig. 7) [41].

The axillary view is shot with the shoulder abducted ideally between 70 and 90 degrees and the beam directed cephalad with the cassette positioned at the superior aspect of the shoulder. It is the best view to image for dislocations and the presence of humeral head compression fractures, glenoid fractures, and fractures of the lesser tuberosity (Fig. 8).

If the patient is unable to tolerate the axillary view because of pain, a Velpeau axillary view can be substituted (see Fig. 8) [41,42]. The patient remains in the shoulder sling and is leaned obliquely backward approximately 30 to 45 degrees over the cassette. The beam is then directed caudally, orthogonal to the cassette. It is beneficial for the surgeon or a trained member of their staff to assist with positioning the arm for accurate imaging with the axillary view. The axillary view is the most frequently omitted image and is a common reason for missed dislocations and fractures [42–44]. With careful positioning of the arm into abduction by the physician, the axillary view can nearly always be obtained [3,10].

The scapular Y view is shot posteroanterior with the beam angled 40 degrees from the coronal plane and is at a right angle from the true AP view. The lateral Y radiograph projects the

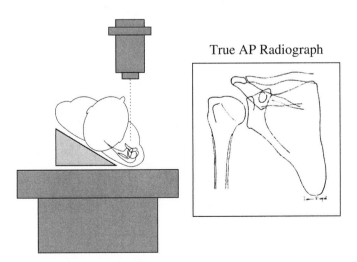

True AP Radiograph

Fig. 7. True anteroposterior radiograph. (*Courtesy of* D. M. Rispoli, MD, Lackland AFB, TX.)

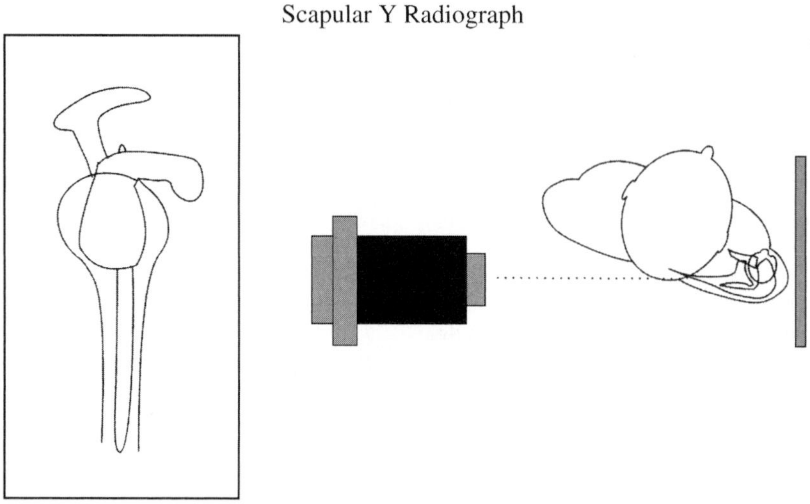

Scapular Y Radiograph

Fig. 8. Valpeau axillary radiograph and axillary radiograph. (*Courtesy of* D. M. Rispoli, MD, Lackland AFB, TX.)

contour of the scapula as the letter Y with the forks of the Y being the body of the scapula in the downward direction, and the upward forks as the coracoid anteriorly, and the spine and the acromion posteriorly. The glenoid is seen at the center of the Y with the humeral head in its reduced position lying at the center of the arms of the Y. In dislocations, the head is seen anterior or posterior to the center of the Y (Fig. 9).

Other radiographic projections are useful for specific fracture types, such as humeral head indentations (so-called Hill-Sachs and reverse

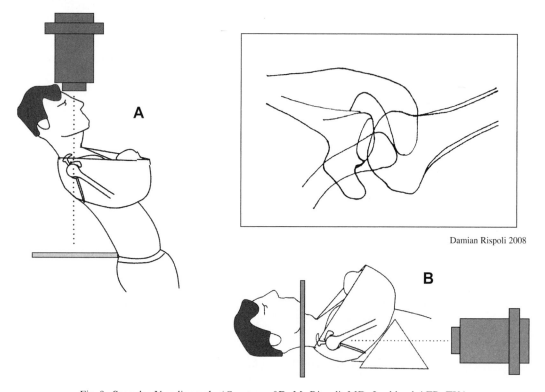

Damian Rispoli 2008

Fig. 9. Scapular Y radiograph. (*Courtesy of* D. M. Rispoli, MD, Lackland AFB, TX.)

Hill-Sachs lesions) or glenoid rim fractures, but are not needed in most cases. The West Point axillary lateral view was initially described by Rokous and colleagues [45] and provides tangential imaging of the anterior glenoid rim. This radiograph is shot with the patient prone with the injured shoulder raised 7 to 8 cm above the table, the head and neck turned away. The cassette is positioned at the superior aspect of the shoulder and the beam is centered at the axilla, 25 degrees inferiorly and 25 degrees medially.

The apical-oblique view is shot with the scapula flat against the cassette while the patient is sitting. The x-ray beam is aimed 45 degrees from the coronal plane and 45 degrees caudally, perpendicular to the cassette and centered on the coracoid. The purpose of this radiograph is to view for posterolateral impression fractures of the humeral head and anterior glenoid rim fractures [41].

The internal rotation view allows for better visualization of the lesser tuberosity. This view may be used in follow-up of a proximal humeral fracture. The internal rotation view is shot with the patient supine. A sandbag is positioned under the elbow placing the humerus horizontal from the top of the table. The arm is abducted and internally rotated 45 degrees with the forearm lying across the trunk. The beam is rotated 15 degrees caudally and is centered over the humeral head [41].

The tangential view is shot with the elbow flexed to 90 degrees, the dorsum of the hand positioned posteriorly to the trunk in the region of the upper lumbar spine, and the thumb pointing upward. The x-ray tube is positioned posterior, lateral, and inferior to the elbow with the cassette placed superiorly to the adducted arm [41].

The Hill-Sachs radiograph is an AP radiograph taken with the humerus in internal rotation revealing posterolateral head impaction fractures [41].

The Stryker notch view is used to evaluate for Hill-Sachs lesions in dislocations and fracture dislocations of the glenohumeral joint. Hall and colleagues [41] first reported a radiograph developed by Stryker called the Stryker notch view. For this radiograph, the patient lies supine with the cassette positioned under the shoulder. The palm of the affected shoulder is placed on the head with the fingers pointed posteriorly and the elbow pointing straight superiorly. The beam is tilted 10 degrees toward the head and is centered over the coracoid.

The Didiee view is an excellent radiographic view for visualization of the anterior inferior glenoid rim; it is shot with the patient prone and the cassette under the shoulder. The forearm is positioned posterior to the trunk and the arm is placed parallel to the top of the table with a 3-in pad under the elbow. The dorsum of the hand is placed on the iliac crest with the thumb pointing upward. In this position the tube is directly lateral to the glenohumeral joint, and the radiograph is shot with the beam angled 45 degrees [41].

CT

CT has enhanced tremendously our ability to image and understand complex proximal humerus fractures. Modern locking-plate technology allows successful internal fixation of complex fracture patterns treated in the past with hemiarthroplasty; CT represents an invaluable tool in the preoperative planning and execution of internal fixation for these complex fractures. The value of CT evaluation has been shown in multiple studies [21,46–48]. Most authors recommend the systematic use of CT scans for preoperative planning, especially for fractures including the greater or lesser tuberosities, humeral head impaction, head splitting, or any other fracture with intra-articular fragments [10,14–16,20,35,37]. The most commonly found occult fractures include lesser tuberosity fractures, head splitting, and posterolateral compression fractures of the humeral head [47].

MRI

Berger and colleagues [49] published several case reports of proximal humerus fractures detected using MRI while investigating for rotator cuff pathologies. These fractures were radiographically occult or showed only subtle abnormalities overlooked on initial reading. Berger concluded that MRI can be a useful diagnostic tool in assessing osseous abnormalities about the proximal humerus potentially leading to improved patient evaluation and treatment. In general, MRI is rarely used in the standard preoperative imaging protocol of proximal humerus fractures.

Summary

The evaluation and treatment of proximal humerus fractures has evolved substantially over the last few decades. The indications for surgery have continued to expand reflecting the increased functional demands of patients and improvements in internal fixation and arthroplasty techniques. The knowledgeable selection of nonoperative treatment, internal fixation, or arthroplasty requires an understanding of the unique features of the different fracture patterns and their natural history. Over time, several classification systems have been proposed to help guide treatment decisions. Most are based on the radiographic appearance of the fracture on plain films, which may be complemented with other imaging studies.

Early classification systems delineated the anatomic components of proximal humeral fractures. Neer developed a classification system based on fracture pathoanatomy that has become convention over the last 40 years. Emphasis on the vascularity of the proximal humerus has led to a deeper understanding of fracture configuration as related to perfusion of the articular segment, and this concept was incorporated into the AO classification system. CT with 3-D reconstruction has allowed recognition of additional fracture lines and patterns and represents an extremely useful tool for the understanding, preoperative planning, and operative execution in the treatment of proximal humerus fractures.

The minimum baseline studies for the evaluation of proximal humerus fractures must include a true AP view of the scapula and glenohumeral joint, an axillary view, and a lateral Y view of the scapula, evaluating the glenohumeral joint and proximal humerus in three perpendicular planes. Alternative radiographic views are helpful for some fractures, such as humeral head indentations and fractures of the glenoid rim. CT is recommended for most proximal humerus fractures, especially when internal fixation is considered. MRI may help identify occult fractures and detect associated rotator cuff tears.

References

[1] Baron JA, Barrett JA, Karagas MR. The epidemiology of peripheral fractures. Bone 1996;18(3 Suppl): 209S–13S.

[2] Codman EA. The shoulder: rupture of the supraspinatus tendon and other lesions in or about the subacromial bursa. Brooklyn (NY): Miller; 1934. p. 262–87.

[3] Neer CS. Displaced proximal humeral fractures. Part I: classification and evaluation. J Bone Joint Surg Am 1970;52:1077–89.

[4] Marsh JL, Slongo T, Agel J, et al. Fracture and dislocation classification compendium—2007. J Orthop Trauma 2007;21(Suppl 10):S1–133.

[5] Edelson G, Kelly I, Vigder F, et al. A three-dimensional classification for fractures of the proximal humerus. J Bone Joint Surg Br 2004;86(3): 413–25.

[6] Dehne E. Fractures at the upper end of the humerus: a classification based on the etiology of trauma. Surg Clin North Am 1945;25:28–47.

[7] Watson-Jones R. Fractures and joint injuries. 4th edition. Baltimore (MD): Williams and Wilkins; 1955.

[8] Bohler L. The treatment of fractures. 5th edition. New York: Grune and Stratton; 1956.

[9] Kocher T. Beitrage zur kenntniss einiger praktisch wichtiger fracturenforamen. Basel and Leipsig: Carl Sollman; 1896.

[10] Neer CS. Four-segment classification of proximal humeral fractures: purpose and reliable use. J Shoulder Elbow Surg 2002;11(4):389–400.

[11] Neer CS II. Shoulder reconstruction. 1st edition. Philadelphia: Saunders; 1990.

[12] Sidor ML, Zuckerman JD, Lyon T, et al. Classification of proximal humeral fractures: the contribution of the scapular, lateral, and axillary radiographs. J Shoulder Elbow Surg 1994;3:24–7.

[13] Mueller ME, Nazarian S, Koch P, et al. The comprehensive classification of fractures of long bones. New York: Springer; 1990. p. 54–63.

[14] Bernstein J, Adler LM, Blank JE, et al. Evaluation of Neer system of classification of proximal humerus fractures with computerized tomographic scans and plain radiographs. J Bone Joint Surg Am 1996;78A:1371–5.

[15] Brorson S, Bagger J, Sylvest A, et al. Improved interobserver variation after training of doctors in the Neer system. J Bone Joint Surg Br 2002;84:950–4.

[16] Kristansen B, Anderson UL, Olsen CA, et al. The Neer classification of fractures of the proximal humerus. An assessment of interobserver variation. Skeletal Radiol 1988;17:420–2.

[17] Sallay PI, Pedowitz RA, Mallon WJ, et al. Reliability and reproducibility of radiographic interpretation of proximal humeral fracture pathoanatomy. J Shoulder Elbow Surg 1997;6:60–9.

[18] Sidor M, Zuckerman J, Lyon T, et al. The Neer classification system for proximal humerus fractures. An assessment of interobserver reliability and intraobserver reproducibility. J Bone Joint Surg Am 1993;75(12):1745–50.

[19] Siebenrock K, Gerber C. The reproducibility of classification of fractures of the proximal end of the humerus. J Bone Joint Surg Am 1993;75(12):1751–5.

[20] Brien H, Noftall F, MacMaster S, et al. Neer's classification system: a critical appraisal. J Trauma 1995;38(2):257–60.

[21] Castagno AA, Shuma WP, Kilcoyne RF, et al. Complex fractures of the proximal humerus: role of CT in treatment. Radiology 1987;165:759–62.

[22] Sjödén GOJ, Movin T, Aspelin P, et al. 3D-radiographic analysis does not improve the Neer and

AO classifications of proximal humeral fractures. Acta Orthop Scand 1999;70(4):325–8.

[23] Sjödén GOJ, Movin T, Günter P, et al. Poor reproducibility of classification of proximal humeral fractures: additional CT of minor value. Acta Orthop Scand 1997;68:239–42.

[24] Guix JMM, Gonzalez AS, Brugalla JV, et al. Proposed protocol for reading images of humeral head fractures. Clin Orthop Relat Res 2006;448:225–33.

[25] Neer CS, Rockwood CA Jr, Bigliani LU, et al. Correspondence. J Bone Joint Surg Am 1994;76:7893.

[26] Resch H, Povacz P, Frohlich R, et al. Percutaneous fixation of three- and four-part fractures of the proximal humerus. J Bone Joint Surg Br 1997;79: 295–300.

[27] Tingart MJ, Apreleva M, von Stechow D, et al. The cortical thickness of the proximal humerus diaphysis predicts bone mineral density of the proximal humerus. J Bone Joint Surg Br 2003;85:611–7.

[28] Nho SJ, Brophy RH, Barker JU, et al. Innovations in the management of displaced proximal humerus fractures. J Am Acad Orthop Surg 2007;15:12–26.

[29] Gardner MJ, Weil Y, Barker JU, et al. The importance of medial support in locked plating of proximal humerus fractures. J Orthop Trauma 2007; 21(3):185–91.

[30] Lee CK, Hansen HR. Post-traumatic avascular necrosis of the humeral head in displaced proximal humeral fractures. J Trauma 1981;21:788–91.

[31] Leysho RL. Closed treatment of fractures of the proximal humerus. Orthop Scand 1984;55:48–51.

[32] Laing PG. The arterial supply of the adult humerus. J Bone Joint Surg Am 1956;38:1105–16.

[33] Gerber C, Schneeberger AG, Vihn TS. The arterial vascularization of the humeral head. An anatomic study. J Bone Joint Surg Am 1990;72:1486–94.

[34] Brooks CH, Revell WJ, Heatley FW. Vascularity of the humeral head after proximal humeral fractures. An anatomical cadaver study. J Bone Joint Surg Br 1993;75:132–6.

[35] Duparc F, Muller J-M, Fréger P. Arterial blood supply to the proximal humeral epiphysis. Surg Radiol Anat 2001;23:185–90.

[36] Meyer C, Alt V, Hassanin H, et al. The arteries of the humeral head and their relevance in fracture treatment. Surg Radiol Anat 2005;27:232–7.

[37] Hertel R, Hempfing A, Stiehler M, et al. Predictors of humeral head ischemia after intracapsular

fracture of the proximal humerus. J Shoulder Elbow Surg 2004;13:427–33.

[38] Jakob RP, Miniaci A, Anson PS, et al. Four-part valgus impacted fractures of the proximal humerus. J Bone Joint Surg Br 1991;73:295–8.

[39] Tamai K, Hamada J, Ohno W, et al. Surgical anatomy of multipart fractures of the proximal humerus. J Shoulder Elbow Surg 2002;11(5):421–7.

[40] Naranja RJ, Ianotti JP. Displaced three- and four-part proximal humeral fractures: evaluation and management. J Am Acad Orthop 2000;8(6):373–82.

[41] Hall R, Isaac F, Booth C. Dislocations of the shoulder with special reference to accompanying small fractures. J Bone Joint Surg 1959;41A:489–94.

[42] Warner JJP, Costouros JG, Gerber C. Fractures of the proximal humerus. In: Bucholz RW, Heckman JD, Court-Brown C, editors. Rockwood and Green's fractures in adults. 6th edition, vol. 1. Philadelphia: Lippincott Williams and Wilkins; 2006. p. 1161–209.

[43] Rowe CR, Zarins B. Chronic unreduced dislocations of the shoulder. J Bone Joint Surg Am 1982;64: 494–505.

[44] Kaar K, Wirth MA, Rockwood CA Jr. Missed posterior fracture-dislocation of the humeral head: a case report with a fifteen-year follow-up after delayed open reduction and internal rotation. J Bone Joint Surg Am 1999;81:708–10.

[45] Rokous JR, Feagin JA, Abbott HG. Modified axillary roentgenogram: a useful adjunct in the diagnosis of recurrent instability of the shoulder. Clin Orthop 1972;82:84–6.

[46] Jurik AG, Albrechtsen J. The use of computed tomography with two- and three-dimensional reconstruction in the diagnosis of three- and four-part fractures of the proximal humerus. Clin Radiol 1994;49:800–4.

[47] Haapamaki VV, Kiuiu MJ, Koskinen SK. Multidetector CT in shoulder fractures. Emerg Radiol 2004; 11:89–94.

[48] Kilcoyne RF, Shuman WP, Matsen FA, et al. The Neer classification of displaced proximal humeral fractures. Spectrum of findings on plain radiographs and CT scans. AJR Am J Roentgenol 1990;15: 1029–33.

[49] Berger P, Ofstein R, Jackson D, et al. MRI demonstration of radiographically occult fractures: What have we been missing? Radiographics 1989;9(3):407–32.

ELSEVIER
SAUNDERS

Orthop Clin N Am 39 (2008) 405–416

ORTHOPEDIC
CLINICS
OF NORTH AMERICA

Percutaneous Fixation of Proximal Humerus Fractures

Brian Magovern, MD[a],*, Matthew L. Ramsey, MD[b]

[a]Shoulder and Elbow Service, Department of Orthopaedic Surgery, Thomas Jefferson University,
925 Chestnut Street, Philadelphia, PA 19107, USA
[b]Rothman Institute, Thomas Jefferson University, 925 Chestnut Street, Philadelphia, PA 19107, USA

Fractures of the proximal humerus are common injuries, accounting for 4% to 5% of all fractures [1]. The incidence sharply increases in the elderly, with 71% of all proximal humerus fractures occurring in patients over the age of 60 years [2,3]. The overall female to male ratio has been reported to be 3:1 but may reach 7:1 in aging populations [2,4]. Moar proximal humerus fractures are minimally displaced and can be treated nonoperatively successfully [5]. A short period of immobilization followed by early motion yields predictably high union rates and good outcomes [2,5–7]. The remaining 15% of proximal humerus fractures are considered displaced. Unless medical contraindications exist, operative management is recommended, because closed treatment of these fractures generally leads to poor results [8,9].

Multiple surgical treatment options have been reported. Traditional techniques include open reduction and internal fixation (ORIF) with plates and screws, and intramedullary, nails, tension-band wiring, and suture fixation [8,10–15]. Arthroscopic assistance has been reported also [16]. Increasing attention has been focused on the importance of careful handling of soft tissues and on the preservation of blood supply during surgical treatment of fractures [17–20]. Although ORIF of proximal humerus fractures may obtain stable fixation and anatomic reduction, significant exposure often is required. Minimally invasive techniques, with less disruption of soft tissue attachments, may offer advantages over conventional fixation. Percutaneous fixation has been described as a viable treatment option for a multitude of fractures in all age groups [21–23]. Closed reduction and percutaneous pinning (CRPP) of the proximal humerus is a less invasive option in selected patients.

CRPP of proximal humerus fractures was reported first by Bohler in 1962 but has received more attention in recent literature [24,25]. The potential advantages compared with ORIF include higher union rates, lower rates of avascular necrosis (AVN), decreased scar formation at the scapulohumeral interface [25], and improved cosmesis. The indications vary depending on fracture type, bone quality, patient factors, and surgeon comfort. This article addresses the indications, biomechanics, surgical technique, and results of percutaneous fixation of proximal humerus fractures.

Codman first noted that the proximal humerus tends to fracture along physeal lines [5]. Four fragments may be created: the shaft, the articular surface, and the greater and lesser tuberosities. Neer [5] based his classification system on these observations. A fragment is considered displaced if it is separated by more than 1 cm or is angulated more than 45°. Although controversy exists regarding the reliability of Neer's classification system [26,27], it remains widely used in both clinical practice and research.

In general, ORIF is recommended for displaced two-part and three-part fractures, and prosthetic replacement is reserved for four-part fractures because of higher rates of AVN. One pattern that deserves special mention is the four-part valgus-impacted fracture. Although technically a four-part fracture according to Neer's criteria, AVN rates have been lower than with displaced four-part fractures, and ORIF may be considered [28].

---

* Corresponding author.
    E-mail address: magovernb@hotmail.com
(B. Magovern).

Indications

Closed reduction and percutaneous fixation may be considered as an alternative to ORIF in selected fractures. Fractures amenable to CRPP include two-part fractures of the surgical neck, greater tuberosity, and lesser tuberosity, three-part surgical neck fractures with involvement of the greater or lesser tuberosity, and valgus-impacted four-part fractures. Fractures of the anatomic neck and head-split fractures generally are not considered for percutaneous fixation.

Closed reduction and percutaneous pinning is a demanding surgical technique. For this technique to be used successfully, several conditions are required: (1) a stable closed reduction, (2) good bone stock, (3) minimal comminution, particularly involving the tuberosity, (4) an intact medial calcar, and (5) a cooperative patient. If acceptable alignment cannot be obtained, the technique should be abandoned in favor of a more traditional open reduction. A limited exposure offers no benefit if the fracture is reduced incompletely, because functional outcome has been shown to correlate with adequacy of reduction and residual deformity [29]. Before draping the extremity, the surgeon may perform an initial closed reduction under image intensification to determine the likelihood of obtaining adequate alignment. Although the final decision is made intraoperatively, the surgeon must have equipment available should ORIF or hemiarthroplasty be required. If an open reduction is necessary, fixation pins still may be placed percutaneously, limiting exposure, as long as the fracture is stable after fixation.

Poor bone quality and fracture comminution are relative contraindications to this technique. Pin loosening and loss of reduction have been attributed to these two factors in several studies [29–31]. CRPP depends on limited fixation, thus requiring excellent bone purchase for support. An intact periosteal sleeve along the medial calcar is thought to be important in providing stability to the fracture and for collateral blood flow to the humeral head [28]. This intact periosteal sleeve probably explains the lower rates of AVN in valgus-impacted four-part fractures compared with other four-part fractures [28,32]. Patients best suited for CRPP have large fracture fragments and good bone stock. Finally, patients must be cooperative and able to comply with the postoperative protocol and rehabilitation.

Biomechanics

Although clinical results have been favorable, biomechanical studies have demonstrated inferior stability with percutaneous pinning compared with other forms of fixation. Wheeler and colleagues [33] created a three-part proximal humerus fracture in a cadaver specimen to compare fixation with an intramedullary nail versus 2.5-mm Schantz pins. The specimens fixed with intramedullary nails were significantly stiffer during cyclic loading and demonstrated higher ultimate loads to failure. Koval and colleagues [34] used a cadaver model to assess stability of 10 different forms of fixation of a simulated two-part surgical neck fracture. Two constructs included 2.5-mm terminally threaded Schantz pins. One configuration placed four pins in parallel passing retrograde into the head from the anterolateral surface of the humerus. The second configuration placed three retrograde pins in a triangular pattern and one antegrade pin through the greater tuberosity. Compared with the T-plate, the two Schantz pin configurations had less resistance to displacement and a lower load to failure in fresh-frozen specimens. When the two Schantz pin groups were compared, the construct with the antegrade pin through the greater tuberosity provided had greater load to failure, suggesting improved stability with biplanar fixation as well as bicortical purchase from one of the pins.

Although percutaneous pinning may be biomechanically less stable than plate and intramedullary nail fixation, certain principles may enhance stability of the construct. Larger-diameter pins offer increased stability. In the study by Koval and colleagues [34], 0.0625 Kirschner wires were included in two of the constructs. Kirschner-wire fixation proved to be biomechanically inferior to 2.5-mm Schantz pins in all aspects of testing. The Kirschner wires also were noted to bend and piston during loading sequences.

Pin configuration has been examined also. Jiang and colleagues [35] demonstrated that pins placed in a parallel pattern provided better torsional stability than pins placed in a convergent pattern. Naidu and colleagues [36] examined four different pin configurations and noted that two lateral pins alone provided the least stability. Torsional stability increased with the addition of an anterior cortical pin, and bending stability increased with the addition of greater tuberosity pins. The authors concluded that biplanar fixation and increasing the number of pins engaging cortex increased stability. Durigan and colleagues [37] compared four different pin configurations using a swine femur model stressed under a varus load. The two constructs that included two antegrade pins through the greater tuberosity had higher loads to failure and less gapping than specimens fixed with only one or with no pins through the tuberosity.

Surgical technique

Preoperative planning

Preoperative evaluation is critical for the success of this technique. A thorough history and physical examination must be performed. The mechanism of injury should be elicited with particular attention to patient-related factors that may have contributed to the fracture. The patient's living situation should be assessed to determine if postoperative needs for activity would preclude CRPP or if the patient's lifestyle raises concerns for the ability to cooperate postoperatively. A careful neurovascular examination is critical, including an assessment of the axillary nerve.

A standard trauma series, including an anteroposterior view of the shoulder perpendicular to the coronal plane and in the plane of the scapula, a lateral view (scapular Y-view), and an axillary view, is obtained. If the patient cannot be positioned for a standard axillary view, a Velpeau axillary view is acceptable [38]. If standard radiographs are not sufficient to appreciate the fracture pattern, CT scan with three-dimensional reconstructions can be very helpful.

Patient positioning

Patient positioning is crucial if this technique is to be used successfully. The surgery can be performed in the supine or beach-chair position, but generally it is easier to perform the surgery with the patient inclined 20° to 30°. The patients should be positioned as far laterally on the table as possible with lateral thorax support to prevent the patient from being pulled off the operating table. The head is immobilized in a head holder. The involved extremity is draped to allow free mobility for reduction maneuvers, fixation, and radiographic imaging (Fig. 1). Image intensification should be positioned to allow complete visualization of the proximal humerus and glenohumeral joint in two orthogonal planes. Placement of a post between the arm and chest

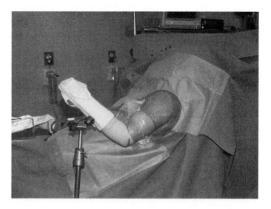

Fig. 1. The patient is positioned in the modified beach-chair position with the affected arm draped free. This position allows intraoperative manipulation of the extremity.

wall may allow the surgeon to lever the shaft laterally to engage the proximal components.

Fracture reduction

The key to minimally invasive techniques is the ability to obtain an anatomic closed reduction. To achieve this goal, it is critical to understand the deforming forces on the fracture fragments. The reduction maneuvers to counteract the deforming forces on the fracture fragments are specific to each fracture pattern. Therefore, fracture-specific methods of reduction are discussed.

If necessary, the fracture fragments can be reduced through a separate small incision made 2 to 3 cm distal to the anterolateral corner of the acromion in line with the anterior aspect of the clavicle (Fig. 2). This technique positions the incision over the region of the surgical neck. This incision also can be used to assist in the reduction of the greater or lesser tuberosity in three- and four-part fractures.

Two-part surgical neck fractures

The major fragments in a two-part surgical neck fracture are the humeral shaft and the humeral head. Because all the rotator cuff attachments to the head fragment are intact, the humeral head typically is in neutral or slight varus position because of unopposed pull of the supraspinatus. The humeral shaft fragment displaces medially and anteriorly and is rotated internally by the pull of the pectoralis major muscle. The humeral head often assumes a retroverted position, not because of muscular pull on the head

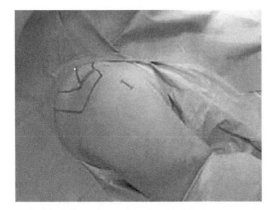

Fig. 2. Accessory reduction portal. This portal assists in reduction of the surgical neck and greater and/or lesser tuberosities. (*From* Keener JD, Parsons BO, Flatow EL, et al. Outcomes after percutaneous reduction and fixation of proximal humerus fractures. J Shoulder Elbow Surg 2007;16:331; with permission).

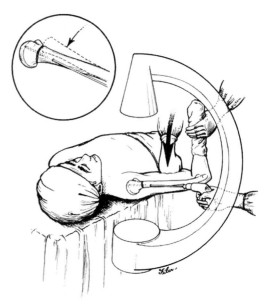

Fig. 3. Longitudinal traction is applied with the arm in abduction. A posteriorly directed force is applied to the humeral shaft reducing the apex anterior angulation of the fracture. (*From* Jaberg H, Warner JJ, Jakob RP. Percutaneous stabilization of unstable fractures of the humerus. J Bone Joint Surg Am 1992;74:509; with permission.)

fragment but because of deformity imposed by the pull of the pectoralis major on the shaft fragment.

The major deforming force is the pectoralis major, and its effects are minimized by flexing, adducting, and internally rotating the humerus. Traction then is applied to the arm, and a posteriorly directed force is applied reducing the apex anterior angulation (Fig. 3). Once reduced, the humerus can be externally rotated to neutral so that the humeral shaft rotationally aligns with the humeral head. The arm can be positioned at the side or in slight abduction, depending on the degree of varus of the humeral head.

Two-part greater and lesser tuberosity fracture

Percutaneous techniques generally are reserved for mobile tuberosity fractures with lesser degrees of displacement. Placement of a percutaneous pin into the tuberosity to hold it in place, followed by rotation of the humerus, may help reduce the tuberosity. Once reduced, a second pin is driven across the fracture site for definitive fixation. Alternatively, tuberosity reduction is accomplished through an incision made 2 to 3 cm distal to the anterolateral acromion in line with the anterior aspect of the clavicle. A reduction pick is introduced, and the tuberosity is reduced and fixed.

If necessary, a small incision off the acromion can be used to introduce a shoulder hook or bone tamp to assist reduction. Percutaneous fixation of lesser tuberosity fractures is used rarely because of the difficulty obtaining reduction and the danger

of injuring neighboring neurovascular structures and fragmenting the tuberosity, which may compromise fixation.

Three-part greater tuberosity fractures

The humeral shaft fragment always assumes a position of anteromedial displacement with slight internal rotation under the influence of the pull of the pectoralis major. The head fragment assumes an internally rotated position because of the unopposed pull of the subscapularis on the intact lesser tuberosity. Reduction of the surgical neck component is performed as described previously. Flexing, adducting, and internally rotating the humerus minimizes the effect of the pectoralis major. Traction then is applied to the arm, and a posteriorly directed force is applied, reducing the apex anterior angulation. Because the humeral head typically is internally rotated, the humeral shaft is maintained in an internally rotated position. The arm is positioned at the side.

Once the surgical neck portion of the fracture is fixed, the arm is positioned in slight external rotation to assist in reduction of the greater tuberosity. The tuberosity is reduced with a reduction hook through the reduction incision previously placed. The greater tuberosity is fixed with antegrade pins or preferably cannulated screws (Fig. 4).

Three-part lesser tuberosity fracture

As noted previously, the humeral shaft fragment assumes a position of anteromedial displacement with slight internal rotation under the influence of the pull of the pectoralis major. The head fragment assumes an abducted, externally rotated, and apex anterior–angulated position because of the unopposed pull of the posterosuperior rotator cuff on the intact greater tuberosity. Reduction of the surgical neck component is performed by flexing and externally rotating the arm. Traction then is applied to the arm, and a posteromedially directed force is applied to the proximal humerus. Because the humeral head typically is externally rotated and abducted, the humeral shaft is externally rotated, and the arm is positioned in abduction once reduction is accomplished. If closed reduction cannot be achieved, placement of a percutaneous awl may help reduce fragments, or Kirschner wires may be used as joysticks to aid reduction [39]. Once the surgical neck portion of the fracture is fixed, the arm is positioned in slight internal rotation to assist in reduction of the lesser tuberosity. The tuberosity is reduced with a reduction hook through the reduction incision previously placed.

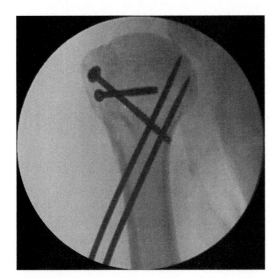

Fig. 4. Fixation of a three-part greater tuberosity fracture. Retrograde anterolateral pins fix the humeral head to the shaft, and cannulated screws fix the tuberosity to the head and shaft.

Four-part valgus-impacted fracture

In the four-part valgus-impacted fracture pattern, the head is centered on the shaft but is impacted into a valgus position. Anatomic reduction of the humeral head is performed by elevating the lateral aspect of the head through the defect between the greater and lesser tuberosity. Because the fracture line between the tuberosities typically occurs slightly posterior to the bicipital groove, a reduction incision can be placed about 2 cm distal to the anterolateral acromion in line with the anterior aspect of the clavicle.

A blunt elevator or small bone tamp is inserted through the tuberosity defect and engages the lateral aspect of the humeral head, disimpacting it from the shaft. The goal of percutaneous reduction is to elevate the lateral aspect of the articular surface hinging on the intact medial periosteum. The head is held in an elevated position while fixation of the head to the shaft is completed.

In some cases, the tuberosities fall back into place into the remaining defect left by the disimpacted articular fragment. This occurrence happens more frequently with the lesser tuberosity. Manual tuberosity reduction may be required in other cases. If required, the greater and lesser tuberosities are reduced with a reduction pick and fixed as necessary (Fig. 5).

Fracture fixation

Fixation of the humeral shaft to the head is performed with terminally threaded 2.5-mm Schantz pins. Other terminally threaded pins that can be used are the guidewires for a 6.5-mm or 7.3-mm cannulated screw set. Terminally threaded pins are preferred because they get purchase in the head fragment, minimizing the risk of pin migration. Smooth Kirschner wires tend to migrate, whereas fully threaded Kirschner wires can wrap up soft tissue inadvertently and therefore are avoided. Several pin positions have been described for fixing the shaft to the humeral head and the tuberosities to the head and shaft (Fig. 6).

Pins to fix the surgical neck portion of the fracture typically are placed in a retrograde fashion from the shaft up into the humeral head. Knowledge of anatomy is critical when using percutaneous techniques. The pins on the lateral cortex should be placed in a safe zone that avoids both the radial and axillary nerves. The radial nerve is relatively protected if pins are kept above

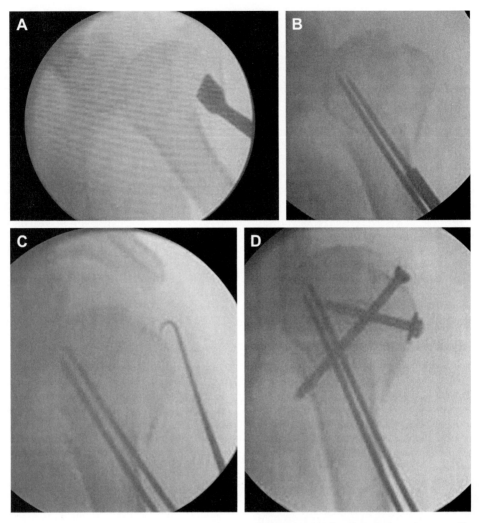

Fig. 5. (*A*) Percutaneous reduction of the humeral head with an elevator placed against the lateral aspect of impacted humeral head. (*B*) Once reduced, the head is stabilized to the shaft with retrograde pins. (*C*) The tuberosity is reduced with external rotation or with the assistance of a reduction too. (*D*) The tuberosity is fixed with cannulated screws. (*From* Keener JD, Parsons BO, Flatow EL, et al. Outcomes after percutaneous reduction and fixation of proximal humerus fractures. J Shoulder Elbow Surg 2007;16:333; with permission.)

the deltoid insertion. The axillary nerve is located an average of 5 cm distal to the acromion; however, it may take a more variable path, particularly the anterior branches [40]. When placing pins through the deltoid, a protective sleeve should be used to decrease the risk of nerve injury. Humeral retroversion averages 19° [41], and percutaneous pins must be directed posteromedially to account for this angle. Pins placed without accounting for retroversion may perforate the articular surface anteriorly while appearing within the bone on anteroposterior imaging.

Anterior pins place the biceps tendon and musculocutaneous nerve at risk.

Several methods are used in attempts to reduce the risk of pin migration. Terminal threads help secure pins in place. Care should be taken to engage dense subchondral bone with the ends of the pins. Penetration of the articular surface followed by retraction may leave a pin with poor purchase that is predisposed to loosening and migration [42]. Last, some authors routinely bend the pins underneath the skin to offer a mechanical block to migration. Unfortunately, as

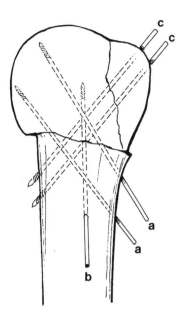

Fig. 6. Terminally threaded pins are placed from the shaft into the head (a) in a retrograde anterolateral position above the deltoid insertion or (b) in a retrograde anterior position. The tuberosity can be fixed with cannulated screws or pins placed (c) in an antegrade lateral position. (*From* Jaberg H, Warner JJ, Jakob RP. Percutaneous stabilization of unstable fractures of the humerus. J Bone Joint Surg Am 1992;74:509; with permission.)

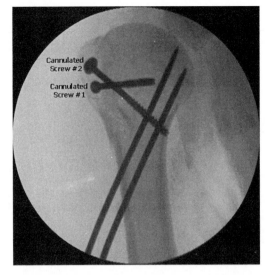

Fig. 7. Tuberosity fixation with 4.5-mm cannulated screws. Initial placement of a horizontal screw (#1) prevents over-reduction of the tuberosity. A second oblique screw is placed that engages the medial cortex at least 2 cm distal to the articular surface.

discussed later, migration still may occur. Depending on bone quality and surgeon preference, pins also may be replaced with cannulated screws. The pins are cut below the surface of the skin but are left prominent enough that they can be palpated once the swelling has subsided. The pins never should be left protruding from the skin because the risk of infection is too great.

Once the humeral head and humeral shaft are fixed, the tuberosities are addressed. Both pin fixation and cannulated screw fixation have been described for securing the tuberosities [25,32]. The authors prefer to use 4.5-mm cannulated screws because they avoid pin irritation against the acromion, which is common with antegrade pins. The guide pin is placed under fluoroscopic guidance. The authors prefer to place the first cannulated screw more horizontally to avoid over-reduction of the tuberosity. The second screw is placed from proximal lateral to distal medial engaging the medial cortex at least 2 cm inferior to the joint surface to minimize the risk of injury to the neurovascular bundle [43] (Fig. 7).

At the conclusion of the case the shoulder is taken through a range of motion under fluoroscopy to evaluate the stability of the construct and to ensure that the pins are not protruding into the joint. Klepps and colleagues [44] evaluated ways to avoid articular penetration based on radiographic criteria. The authors divided the proximal humerus into three zones on the anteroposterior and axillary views. Posterior wire penetration was the most difficult to detect and was seen best with the humerus in 60° of external rotation to compensate for humeral retroversion.

Postoperative management

The arm is immobilized in a sling for the first few weeks postoperatively. The patient is permitted immediate elbow, wrist, and hand motion. If the tuberosities are fixed with cannulated screws instead of antegrade pins, pendulum exercises can begin immediately if fixation is thought to be adequate. Pins placed to fix the tuberosities generally are removed at 3 to 4 weeks, and the retrograde pins are removed 4 to 6 weeks after surgery (Fig. 8).

Patients need to be followed closely in the postoperative period. Until the pins are removed, radiographs should be taken weekly to be sure reduction is maintained and pin migration has not

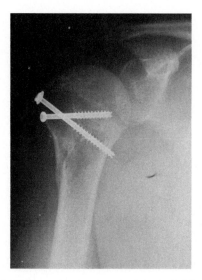

Fig. 8. Radiographic appearance of the healed fracture following pin removal.

occurred. Pin migration may necessitate early removal.

Progressive active-assisted range of motion is begun following pin removal once fracture healing is demonstrated radiographically. The authors tend to delay strengthening exercises until fracture union is complete and range of motion is progressing nicely, which typically takes about 12 weeks.

Complications

Pin migration

Pin migration is a frequent problem around the shoulder and can have disastrous consequences. Although the cause remains unknown, pins placed around the shoulder have a propensity for migration. First reported by Mazet [45] in 1943, many factors, including respiratory motions, increased mobility of the upper extremity, and regional resorption of bone, have been theorized to play a role in the cause. The incidence is believed to be underreported secondary to its dramatic nature and its potential legal ramifications. Lyons and Rockwood [46] reviewed 37 reports that included 47 instances of pin migration when used around the shoulder girdle. Seventeen pins migrated to major vascular structures including the heart, subclavian artery, ascending aorta, and pulmonary artery. Eight pins migrated to the lung, 10 to the mediastinum, and five to the cervical spine. One

pin migrated to the trachea and was coughed up by the patient. Pin migration was not limited to the chest: one migrated to the retroperitoneum, one to the spleen, and one to the right orbit causing a painful exophthalmos. Eight patients died, six of whom died suddenly of catastrophic cardiovascular events. Most events occurred by eight months postoperatively, but earlier migration occurs frequently. Mellado and colleagues [30] reported a case of intrathoracic migration of pins placed for a proximal humeral fracture 10 days after surgery, despite the pins having been bent under the skin. One pin was believed to penetrate lung parenchyma contributing to a hemothorax.

Despite precautionary measures, such as using terminally threaded pins bent under the skin, migration still occurs. Close follow-up is mandatory. Patients must be counseled on the importance of postoperative compliance and symptoms of concern. Immediate postoperative radiographs should be taken to document position, and pins should be removed if there is any change on subsequent films or evidence of loosening.

Infection

Although any implanted hardware may become infected, pins left protruding from the skin are at particularly high risk. Superficial infections generally are treated with local wound care, pin removal, and oral antibiotics. Deeper infections are less common but can lead to significant complications including osteomyelitis of the humerus (Fig. 9). For this reason, pins never should be left protruding from the skin. Patients at higher risk for infection, such as those who have diabetes or immunosuppression, should be monitored closely, and any suspicion of infection should be treated aggressively.

Loss of fixation/malunion/non-union

Union rates following CRPP reportedly are high, probably secondary to the lack of soft tissue dissection required for reduction and fixation. More commonly, loss of fixation and malunion occur. Patients at increased age who have osteoporosis and those who have fracture comminution are at higher risk. Early pin loosening and loss of fixation should be recognized, because surgical correction still may be possible. Depending on the degree of loss of fixation, revision CRPP or ORIF should be performed.

Malunion has been defined in several different ways, making it challenging to compare patients

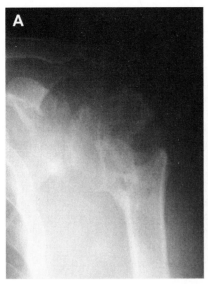

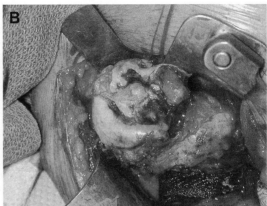

Fig. 9. (*A*) Radiograph and (*B*) intraoperative photograph of a patient who has osteomyelitis of the humeral head with bone destruction from pins left protruding from the skin.

across studies. The most common residual deformities include varus angulation of the head and posterosuperior displacement of the greater tuberosity. Functional loss and pain may result. Radiographic deformity, however, may be surprisingly well tolerated by the patient, and this tolerability should be kept in mind in considering an extensive osteotomy procedure.

Avascular necrosis

The development of AVN is determined largely by the injury itself and not necessarily by the course of treatment [47]. There are, however, suggestions that the rate of AVN is lower with CRPP than with ORIF [48]. The main arterial supply to the humeral head is from the arcuate branch of the anterior circumflex humeral artery, which courses along the lateral edge of the bicipital groove [49]. This structure may be violated by plates placed during open procedures. Although the rate may be lower after CRPP, AVN does occur. In the study by Jaberg and colleagues [24], AVN developed in two distinct forms. One group developed localized areas of AVN with cystosclerotic changes; in the other group the articular surface collapsed completely. The group that had localized changes had gradual resolution of pain and radiographic changes and had no further treatment; the group that had more severe involvement required hemiarthroplasty. The

changes of AVN may take as long as 2 years to develop, and patients should be followed for that length of time.

Neurovascular injury

Despite the lack of exposure and the relative proximity of vital structures, neurovascular injury fortunately is very uncommon with CRPP. Several cadaveric studies have examined the relationship of neurovascular structures to percutaneously placed pins, revealing the potential danger of the procedure. Kamineni and colleagues [50] performed percutaneous pinning on 40 specimens using the technique described by Jaberg and colleagues [24]. Three injuries to the axillary nerve were noted: two direct penetrations and one injury to perineural tissue. No injuries to the circumflex humeral vessels occurred. Rowles and colleagues [43] performed percutaneous pinning in 10 cadavers to examine the proximity of neurovascular structures. Seven of 10 proximal lateral pins were located within 2 mm from the axillary nerve. Of 10 anterior pins, 1 pierced the cephalic vein, and 2 penetrated the biceps tendon. In 2 of 10 specimens, the greater tuberosity pins tented the neurovascular bundle after passing through the medial cortex. Based on these studies, it is clear that neurovascular structures are at risk during CRPP, and a thorough knowledge of the anatomy is mandatory.

Outcomes

Although no head-to-head studies have compared percutaneous pinning and other forms of treatment, the results of CRPP have been favorable. Several large series have examined the outcomes after percutaneous fixation of proximal humerus fractures. Jaberg and colleagues [24] presented the first large series of adults treated with CRPP. Forty-eight patients were followed for an average of 3 years. Seventy percent of patients achieved a good or excellent result. Four patients had a severe loss of reduction. Revision CRPP led to a good or excellent result in all four patients. Two patients developed pseudarthroses believed to be secondary to metaphyseal comminution. The remaining 48 fractures united by 8 weeks. Five patients developed infections, four of whom were treated with pin removal and local care. One diabetic patient developed a deep infection requiring multiple debridements and partial humeral head resection. Two patients who had fractures involving the anatomic neck developed complete articular collapse secondary to AVN and eventually underwent hemiarthroplasty.

More recently, in a multicenter study, Keener and colleagues [25] examined 27 patients treated with CRPP with an average follow-up of 35 months. There were seven two-part, eight three-part, and 12 four-part fractures. All of the four-part fractures were classified as valgus impacted. Patients averaged 142° of elevation and 51° of external rotation at final follow-up. The mean visual analogue scale (VAS) for pain was 1.4 on a scale of 1 to 10. The mean American Shoulder and Elbow Surgeons' (ASES) score was 83.4, and the mean Constant score was 73.9 with no significant differences based on age or fracture pattern. All achieved radiographic union by 3 months. Malunion, defined as a neck shaft angle less than 120° or greater than 150°, tuberosity displacement greater than 5 mm, or a position of the greater tuberosity less than 2 mm or more than 10 mm below the articular margin, was seen in 17% of patients. Although numbers were small, there was no difference in VAS, ASES, or Constant scores between those patients who did or did not develop a malunion. One four-part fracture developed whole-head collapse secondary to AVN by 9 months postoperatively. No infections occurred. One pin was removed for loosening, and the fracture healed in a varus position.

In a study evaluating only three- and four-part fractures, Resch and colleagues [32] examined 27 patients after CRPP. Nine patients had three-part fractures, and 18 had four-part fractures. Age- and gender-adjusted Constant scores for the three- and four-part fractures were 91% and 87%, respectively. All patients who were working preoperatively resumed their previous employment. Fenichel and colleagues [31] reported 70% good or excellent results in 56 patients after CRPP. The Constant score averaged 81. All achieved union with no evidence of AVN. Herscovici and colleagues [42] treated 47 patients who had 49 fractures of the proximal humerus with CRPP using differing hardware. Of the three-part fractures, all of those fixed with Kirschner wires had failure of fixation. Four patients had four-part fractures and had uniformly poor results. Three developed AVN, and one healed with a 70° varus deformity.

Summary

Surgical reduction and fixation is recommended for displaced two- and three-part fractures and for valgus-impacted four-part fractures. Closed reduction and percutaneous pinning may offer advantages over conventional fixation techniques. Potential benefits include higher union rates, decreased AVN, decreased scarring, and improved cosmesis. Despite favorable clinical results, biomechanical studies have shown that pinning constructs are less stable than plate and intramedullary nail fixation. Larger-diameter pins, such as 2.5-mm Schanz pins, and configurations with biplanar fixation and bicortical purchase from greater tuberosity pins improve stability.

Closed reduction aims to counter the pull of deforming muscle units. Longitudinal traction, slight abduction, and internal rotation reduce the shaft to the proximal segment. Two 2.5-mm terminally threaded Schantz pins are placed lateral to medial, accounting for humeral retroversion. One pin is placed from the anterior cortex for added stability. Tuberosity reduction may require a small incision to introduce an awl or shoulder hook. Two further pins are placed through the greater tuberosity obtaining bicortical purchase in the medial shaft. Pins may be replaced with cannulated screws or bent under the skin to decrease the risk of hardware migration. Potential complications include pin migration, infection, AVN, neurovascular injury, and malunion. Clinical outcomes have been comparable with conventional techniques, with studies reporting approximately 70% good to excellent results. Although no comparative studies exist, CRPP is a safe and effective procedure that offers significant potential advantages in the treatment of proximal humerus fractures.

References

[1] Buhr AJ, Cooke AM. Fracture patterns. Lancet 1959;1:531–6.

[2] Lind T, Kroner K, Jensen J. The epidemiology of fractures of the proximal humerus. Arch Orthop Trauma Surg 1989;108:285–7.

[3] Horak J, Nilsson BE. Epidemiology of fracture of the upper end of the humerus. Clin Orthop 1975; 112:250–3.

[4] Rose SH, Melton J, Morrey BF, et al. Epidemiologic features of humeral fractures. Clin Orthop 1982;168: 24–30.

[5] Neer CS. Displaced proximal humeral fractures: part I. classification and evaluation. J Bone Joint Surg Am 1970;52:1077–89.

[6] Koval KJ, Gallagher MA, Marsicano JG, et al. Functional outcome after minimally displaced fractures of the proximal part of the humerus. J Bone Joint Surg Am 1997;79:203–7.

[7] Tejwani NC, Liporace F, Walsh M, et al. Functional outcome following one-part proximal humeral fractures: a prospective study. J Shoulder Elbow Surg 2008;17:216–9.

[8] Neer CS. Displaced proximal humeral fractures: part II. Treatment of three-part and four-part displacement. J Bone Joint Surg Am 1970;52:1090–103.

[9] Leyshon RL. Closed treatment of fractures of the proximal humerus. Acta Orthop Scand 1984;55: 48–51.

[10] Kristiansen B, Christiansen SW. Plate fixation of proximal humeral fractures. Acta Orthop Scand 1986;57:320–3.

[11] Hawkins RJ, Bell RH, Gurr K. The three-part fracture of the proximal part of the humerus. J Bone Joint Surg Am 1986;68:1410–4.

[12] Cuomo F, Flatow EL, Maday MG, et al. Open reduction and internal fixation of two- and three-part displaced surgical neck fractures of the proximal humerus. J Shoulder Elbow Surg 1992;1: 287–95.

[13] Flatow EL, Cuomo F, Maday MG, et al. Open reduction and internal fixation of two-part displaced fractures of the greater tuberosity of the proximal part of the humerus. J Bone Joint Surg Am 1991; 73:1213–8.

[14] Banco SP, Andrisani D, Ramsey M, et al. The parachute technique: valgus impaction osteotomy for two-part fractures of the surgical neck of the humerus. J Bone Joint Surg Am 2001;83:S38–42.

[15] Williams GR, Wong KL. Two-part and three-part fractures: open reduction versus closed reduction and percutaneous pinning. Orthop Clin North Am 2000;31:1–21.

[16] Taverna E, Sansone V, Battistella F. Arthroscopic treatment for greater tuberosity fractures: rationale and surgical technique. Arthroscopy 2004;20:53–7.

[17] Schandelmaier P, Partenheimer A, Koenemann B, et al. Distal femoral fractures and LISS stabilization. Injury 2001;32(S3):SC55–63.

[18] Fankhauser F, Gruber G, Schippinger G, et al. Minimal-invasive treatment of distal femoral fractures with the LISS (Less Invasive Stabilization System): a prospective study of 30 fractures with a follow up of 20 months. Acta Orthop Scand 2004;75:55–60.

[19] Anglen J, Choi L. Treatment options in pediatric femoral shaft fractures. J Orthop Trauma 2005;19: 724–33.

[20] Boldin C, Fankhauser F, Hofer HP, et al. Three-year results of proximal tibia fractures treated with the LISS. Clin Orthop 2006;445:222–9.

[21] Koval K, Sanders R, Borelli J, et al. Indirect reduction and percutaneous screw fixation of displaced tibial plateau fractures. J Orthop Trauma 1992;6: 340–6.

[22] Paradis G, Lavallee P, Gagnon N, et al. Supracondylar fractures of the humerus in children. Technique and results of crossed percutaneous K-wire fixation. Clin Orthop 1993;297:231–7.

[23] Kofoed H, Alberts A. Femoral neck fractures. 165 Cases treated by multiple percutaneous pinning. Acta Orthop Scand 1980;51:127–36.

[24] Jaberg H, Warner JJ, Jakob RP. Percutaneous stabilization of unstable fractures of the humerus. J Bone Joint Surg Am 1992;74:508–15.

[25] Keener JD, Parsons BO, Flatow EL, et al. Outcomes after percutaneous reduction and fixation of proximal humerus fractures. J Shoulder Elbow Surg 2007;16:330–8.

[26] Sidor ML, Zuckerman JD, Lyon T, et al. The Neer classification system for proximal humeral fractures. An assessment of interobserver reliability and intraobserver reproducibility. J Bone Joint Surg Am 1993;75:1745–50.

[27] Siebenrock KA, Gerber C. The reproducibility of classification of fractures of the proximal end of the humerus. J Bone Joint Surg Am 1993;75:1751–5.

[28] Jakob RP, Miniaci A, Anson PS, et al. Four-part valgus impacted fractures of the proximal humerus. J Bone Joint Surg Br 1991;73:295–8.

[29] Calvo E, de Miguel I, de la Cruz J, et al. Percutaneous fixation of displaced proximal humeral fractures: indications based on the correlation between clinical and radiographic results. J Shoulder Elbow Surg 2007;16:774–81.

[30] Mellado JM, Calmet J, Forcada IL, et al. Early intrathoracic migration of Kirschner wires used for percutaneous osteosynthesis of a two-part humeral neck fracture: a case report. Emerg Radiol 2004;11:49–52.

[31] Fenichel I, Oran A, Burstein G, et al. Percutaneous pinning using threaded pins as a treatment option for unstable two- and three-part fractures of the proximal humerus: a retrospective study. Int Orthop 2006;30:153–7.

[32] Resch H, Povacz P, Frohlich R, et al. Percutaneous fixation of three- and four-part fractures of the proximal humerus. J Bone Joint Surg Br 1997;79: 295–300.

[33] Wheeler D, Colville MR. Biomechanical comparison of intramedullary and percutaneous pin fixation for proximal humeral fracture fixation. J Orthop Trauma 1997;11:363–7.

[34] Koval K, Blair B, Takei R, et al. Surgical neck fractures of the proximal humerus: a laboratory evaluation of ten fixation techniques. J Trauma 1996;40:778–83.

[35] Jiang C, Zhu Y, Wang M, et al. Biomechanical comparison of different pin configurations during percutaneous pinning for the treatment of proximal humerus fractures. J Shoulder Elbow Surg 2007;16: 235–9.

[36] Naidu SH, Bixler B, Capo JT, et al. Percutaneous pinning of proximal humerus fractures: a biomechanical study. Orthopedics 1997;20: 1073–6.

[37] Durigan A, Barbieri CH, Mazzer N, et al. Two-part surgical neck fractures of the humerus: mechanical analysis of the fixation with four Schantz-type threaded pins in four different assemblies. J Shoulder Elbow Surg 2005;14:96–102.

[38] Bloom MH, Obata WG. Diagnosis of posterior dislocation of the shoulder with use of Velpeau axillary and angle-up roentgenographic views. J Bone Joint Surg Am 1967;49:943–9.

[39] Chen C, Chao E, Tu Y, et al. Closed management and percutaneous fixation of unstable proximal humerus fractures. J Trauma 1998;45:1039–45.

[40] Burkhead W, Scheinberg R, Box G. Surgical anatomy of the axillary nerve. J Shoulder Elbow Surg 1992;1:31–6.

[41] Robertson DD, Yuan J, Bigliani LU, et al. Three-dimensional analysis of the proximal part of the humerus: relevance to arthroplasty. J Bone Joint Surg Am 2000;82:1594–602.

[42] Herscovici D, Saunders DT, Johnson MP, et al. Percutaneous fixation of proximal humeral fractures. Clin Orthop 2000;375:97–104.

[43] Rowles DJ, McGrory JE. Percutaneous pinning of the proximal part of the humerus: an anatomic study. J Bone Joint Surg Am 2001;82:1695–9.

[44] Klepps SJ, Miller SL, Lin J, et al. Determination of radiographic guidelines for percutaneous pinning of proximal humerus fractures using a cadaveric model. Orthopedics 2007;30:636–41.

[45] Mazet R. Migration of a Kirschner wire from the shoulder region into the lung: report of two cases. J Bone Joint Surg Am 1943;25:477–83.

[46] Lyons FA, Rockwood CA. Migration of pins used in operations on the shoulder. J Bone Joint Surg Am 1990;72:1262–7.

[47] Hertel R, Hempfing A, Stiehler M, et al. Predictors of humeral head ischemia after intracapsular fracture of the proximal humerus. J Shoulder Elbow Surg 2004;13:427–33.

[48] Kralinger F, Irenberger A, Lechner C, et al. Vergleich der offenen vs. perkutanen Versorgung der Oberarmkopffraktur [Comparison of open versus percutaneous treatment for humeral head fracture]. Unfallchirurg 2006;109:406–10.

[49] Gerber C, Schneeberger AG, Vinh TS. The arterial vascularization of the humeral head: an anatomical study. J Bone Joint Surg Am 1990;72:1486–94.

[50] Kamineni S, Ankem H, Sanghavi S. Anatomical considerations for percutaneous proximal humeral fracture fixation. Injury 2004;35:1133–6.

ELSEVIER
SAUNDERS

Orthop Clin N Am 39 (2008) 417–428

ORTHOPEDIC
CLINICS
OF NORTH AMERICA

Locked Intramedullary Nailing for Treatment of Displaced Proximal Humerus Fractures

Allan A. Young, MBBS, MSpMed, PhD[a],
Jeffery S. Hughes, MBBS, FRACS, FAOrthA[b],*

[a]Department of Orthopaedic and Traumatic Surgery, Royal North Shore Hospital,
Pacific Highway, St. Leonards, Sydney, NSW 2065, Australia
[b]Sydney Shoulder and Elbow Associates, Level 1, The Gallery, 445 Victoria Avenue, Chatswood,
Sydney, NSW 2067, Australia

Management of displaced proximal humerus fractures remains a challenge despite significant advances in our understanding of the pathoanatomy of the injury and modern innovations in treatment modalities. The natural history of nondisplaced fractures suggests that nonoperative management is appropriate in these situations; however, the outcome of such conservative management for displaced or unstable fracture patterns has not been so favorable with persistent pain, stiffness, and dysfunction [1,2]. The literature is deficient in high-level randomized prospective controlled studies to provide definitive guidance on appropriate management [2,3]; however, surgical intervention is generally recommended for displaced proximal humerus fractures, especially if the patient can participate in a rigorous rehabilitation program.

Surgical management of displaced proximal humeral fractures consists of either humeral head preservation by a range of osteosynthesis techniques or, alternatively, salvage with hemiarthroplasty. Controversy surrounds the optimal technique for fixation of displaced fractures, although locked intramedullary nailing is emerging as a preferred technique in managing displaced proximal humerus fractures in appropriately selected patients. This technique provides stable fracture fixation allowing early postoperative mobilization critical in ensuring a pain-free

shoulder with a functional range of motion. Additional advantages include the ability to insert by way of a minimally invasive approach with limited soft tissue dissection, achieve accurate anatomic reduction, provide a secure construct even in the situation of osteopenic bone or comminution, and manage fractures of the proximal humerus extending into the shaft (Fig. 1).

Design of locked intramedullary nails used for fixation of proximal humerus fractures

Intramedullary fixation is commonly used to treat various long bone fractures and has become the standard of care for most diaphyseal and selected metaphyseal injuries in the lower extremity [4]. Intramedullary nails are load-sharing devices with reduced lever arms for fragmentary fixation. Although traditional intramedullary nails failed to adequately control metaphyseal fragments, modern implants allow for stable fixation of complex fracture patterns effectively resisting bending and torsional moments [5–7]. Most current intramedullary nails are made from titanium alloys. Locking of the nail allows for control of rotation and prevents migration of the implant.

Implant considerations

Intramedullary nails designed specifically for proximal humerus fixation incorporate multiple proximal locking screws with multiplanar configurations. This allows independent fixation of the greater and lesser tuberosities to the humeral head fragment, which then provides the ability to

* Corresponding author.
  E-mail address: jshughes@sydneyortho.com.au
(J.S. Hughes).

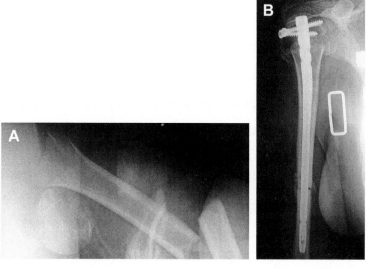

Fig. 1. A high-energy motor vehicle collision resulted in a segmental humeral fracture with a proximal humeral component (*A*). Open reduction and internal fixation with an intramedullary nail allowed rigid fixation with a less invasive surgical exposure (*B*).

control rotational, longitudinal, and angular instability (Fig. 2). Optimal screw positions and angles have been determined based on typical proximal humeral dimensions to treat the most common fracture patterns and to ensure that the screws are in the best-quality bone in the humeral head and avoid the axillary nerve. Alternate oblique holes allow placement of cortical screws to achieve fixation in the medial metaphyseal region.

Additional stability of the tuberosity fragments can be obtained by anchoring sutures to the locking screws. Radiolucent targeting guides, for screw insertion, are used with most systems. Proximal locking screws that thread into the nail have been developed to create a fixed-angle device and to prevent backing out of screws, a problem with earlier designs. Some nails also come with a proximal humeral blade option (Expert Proximal

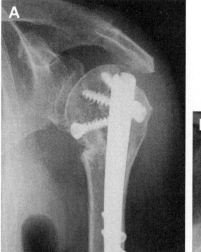

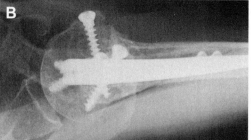

Fig. 2. An elderly active patient presented with a four-part proximal humerus fracture. Intraoperatively it was reducible and was fixed with a locked intramedullary nail (*A*). The fracture headed without avascular necrosis (*B*).

Humeral Nail, Synthes, Pennsylvania, USA) with angular locking designed for a better hold and higher stability, especially in osteoporotic bone. Straighter nails (Trigen, Smith and Nephew, Tennessee, USA; Targon PH, Aesculap, Tuttlingen, Germany) allow for a medialized entry point thereby avoiding potential fracture extension from tuberosity fractures and resultant loss of stability. Most currently available intramedullary nails are cannulated and can be inserted with an unreamed or reamed technique. Proximal humeral nails can also be dynamized as desired. Most fracture patterns are amenable to treatment with standard length nails (eg, the Polarus Nail [Acumed, Hillsboro, Oregon, USA] is 150 mm long). Longer nails are available with most systems and are useful in certain situations, such as when fractures extend into the metadiaphyseal region, are segmental, or are pathologic secondary to metastatic disease.

Patient selection and preoperative planning

As for other techniques of osteosynthesis, the decision to proceed with locked intramedullary nailing depends on numerous factors related to the patient, the surgeon, and the pattern of injury. The patient's age, bone quality, activity level, arm dominance, expectations, and ability to comply with postoperative rehabilitation must be taken into consideration, in addition to the presence of medical comorbidities that may preclude surgical intervention. With respect to the pattern of injury, three specific aspects must be assessed: (1) head vascularity, (2) orientation of the tuberosities relative to the head, and (3) stability of the head complex relative to the shaft.

Head vascularity

Perfusion of the humeral head is an important factor influencing the decision to proceed with osteosynthesis. The presence of head ischemia has been associated with worse outcomes following surgical fixation of proximal humerus fractures [8,9]. Radiographic criteria have been established by Hertel and colleagues [10] to predict the vascularity of the humeral head, the most relevant predictors of ischemia being the length of the posteromedial metaphyseal head extension, the integrity of the medial hinge, and the basic fracture type. In the presence of a metaphyseal extension or medial hinge, the humeral head is likely to survive and internal fixation is a reasonable choice most of the time. In the absence of these positive predictive factors other aspects, such as the patient's age and bone quality, need to be considered before embarking on osteosynthesis.

In an elderly individual who has osteopenic bone and an avascular head, hemiarthroplasty offers a "one-operation" solution and can be expected to provide satisfactory pain relief, although with a variable functional outcome [11–14]. In a young patient who has good quality bone, however, head preservation is a priority regardless of the fracture pattern or likelihood of ischemia. Previous reports have demonstrated that satisfactory outcomes can be expected in the setting of avascular necrosis provided fracture reduction is anatomic and maintained until union [15,16]. Furthermore, collapse of the humeral head in patients who have avascular necrosis can potentially be avoided by administration of an osteoclast inhibitor, such as Zoledronate (J.S. Hughes, unpublished data, 2005); however, further work is required to better delineate this approach.

Tuberosity/head orientation

Displacement of tuberosity fragments in proximal humerus fractures occurs in predictable patterns based on deforming muscular forces. Tendinous insertions of supraspinatus, infraspinatus, and teres minor muscles act on the greater tuberosity to displace it in a posterior, superior, and medial direction. In active patients who have expectations of a good functional outcome, reduction is recommended for fragments with displacement of 5 mm or greater [17,18]. Similarly, fractures of the lesser tuberosity that tend to retract medially from the pull of the subscapularis muscle need to be reduced and fixed. In isolated fractures of the greater or lesser tuberosities requiring reduction, limited internal fixation is usually recommended with sutures or screws, or a combination of both [17,18]. When these fractures occur in combination with a fracture of the surgical neck, the head fragment often tilts into varus with a medially displaced shaft. To achieve the best functional outcomes for patients in this scenario, the goal of operative fixation is anatomic reduction of the head complex [8,19].

Head complex/shaft stability

Following a determination that the head/ tuberosity orientation can be restored, the stability of the head complex relative to the shaft must be addressed. The medial periosteal hinge is essential in providing support and loss of this anatomic restraint results in longitudinal, rotational, and angular instability. In unstable fracture patterns the head tends to assume an extension deformity relative to the medially displaced shaft. Operative intervention must aim to correct such deformities and provide stable anatomic fixation of the head complex to the shaft. In situations in which this hinge remains intact, as in the valgus impacted four-part fracture pattern, the head complex is able to be impacted onto the shaft with stability following tuberosity reduction and limited fixation may be all that is required.

Based on these considerations, a treatment algorithm has been devised for managing proximal humerus fractures Table 1. Locked intramedullary nailing is recommended for treatment of displaced fractures in which the head/tuberosity orientation can be restored but the head complex remains unstable relative to the shaft. Avascular necrosis remains a concern in these cases as

a consequence of at-risk blood supply to the humeral head during the initial injury, fracture manipulation, and surgical exposure. Meticulous surgical technique and minimal soft tissue dissection are highly desirable to reduce the risk for avascular necrosis and intramedullary nailing is superior to plate fixation in that respect.

The technique of intramedullary nailing is also particularly useful in patients who have fracture extension into the shaft, a finding supported by others [20]. The technique is similarly useful in segmental fractures and pathologic fractures secondary to metastatic disease. It is therefore recommended that even those surgeons favoring alternative treatment methods for proximal humerus fractures should familiarize themselves with the technique of intramedullary nailing, which can be of value in these specific situations.

In some cases, where interpretation of the fracture pattern is difficult based on routine plain radiographic trauma series, including an

Table 1

Algorithm for the management of proximal humerus fractures

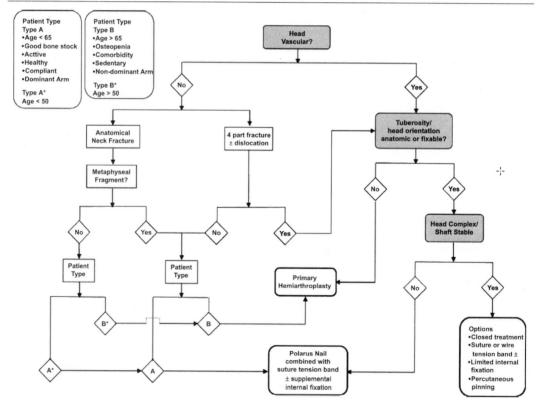

anteroposterior view of the glenohumeral joint, a scapular lateral view, and an axillary view, we recommend obtaining CT scans. Three-dimensional CT reconstructions provide a better appreciation of tuberosity displacement and comminution, in addition to the position of the head fragment relative to the shaft. Regardless of the preoperative planning measures outlined previously, we often make the final decision to proceed with intramedullary fixation in the operating theater. A definitive assessment can be made of head/tuberosity orientation and head complex/shaft stability after the fracture is manipulated under fluoroscopy.

Surgical technique

The patient is placed in a beach-chair position with the shoulder over the edge of the table. Intraoperative fluoroscopy is used and the setup of this should be checked before draping the patient to ensure unimpeded access during the case. The fracture is then manipulated under fluoroscopic control and an assessment of fracture stability used to guide decision making as described previously.

The choice of surgical approach depends on the type of fracture. Although two-part surgical neck fractures are best treated by closed nailing and a limited anterior deltoid splitting approach to allow for nail insertion, most three- and four-part fracture patterns require open reduction by way of a deltopectoral approach. During this approach, a large fracture hematoma is usually encountered and needs to be removed to better visualize the underlying anatomy. Soft tissue stripping is kept to a minimum while exposing the fracture to preserve the remaining vascularity of the humeral head. Exposure is facilitated by placing a Browne retractor beneath the deltoid muscle. The deltoid insertion must be preserved and care needs to be taken during the dissection and retraction. Heavy sutures (#5 Ethibond) are placed at the bone–tendon junction of the teres minor/infraspinatus, supraspinatus, and subscapularis, which allows for subsequent control of the tuberosities during reduction and fixation. The rotator interval is then opened to allow an intra-articular inspection/palpation and assessment of the humeral head position and integrity and later to avoid implant perforation of the joint surface.

Reduction and fixation then proceeds in an ordered sequence as previously outlined, initially addressing the tuberosity/head orientation, followed by stabilization of the head complex to the shaft. Essentially, the goal is to convert a four-part fracture into a three-part fracture, a three-part fracture into a two-part fracture, and so on. The first step is reduction of the head fragment. The reduction maneuver is performed according to the direction of head displacement, which is usually in one of two positions: valgus and extension, or varus and flexion. Under image intensification, a bone tamp is used to push on a specific quadrant of the peripheral aspect of the head fragment to effect the reduction in both planes (eg, if the head is in valgus and extension the posterior superior quadrant is elevated), while at the same time anatomic reduction is achieved by balancing the tension in the superior, posterior, and anterior traction sutures (Fig. 3). These sutures are grasped together and pulled laterally thereby forming a conelike configuration. The center of rotation of this laterally directed reduction force applied to the tuberosities therefore coincides with the center of the humeral head. It is important also that the head segment is not overreduced. The head complex, consisting of the head fragment and both tuberosities, can then be provisionally fixed with Kirschner wires. These Kirschner wires must be placed sufficiently anterior and posterior in the head complex using the greater and lesser tuberosity corridors, so as not to interfere with insertion of the nail. A final decision to proceed with intramedullary nail fixation can now be made based on the stability of the head complex in relation to the shaft. If the fracture pattern is stable, then limited fixation with screw or tension band sutures may be all that is required. In the presence of significant medial periosteal stripping, however, the head and shaft cannot be stably impacted and intramedullary nailing is required.

The key to intramedullary fixation is the correct entry site. An accurate insertion site provides a good approximation of varus/valgus alignment of the shaft. This site should be a point 1 cm posterior to the anterior edge of the supraspinatus and at the junction of the greater tuberosity and articular cartilage. Occasionally, a fracture line through the tuberosity is at this point and the head segment may need to be notched. A 1-cm longitudinal split is made in the supraspinatus tendon and an awl is used to make a provisional hole at the entry site. This hole is usually enlarged with an opening drill of appropriate size relative to the nail, particularly in younger patients who have hard bone. The head complex and shaft are manually reduced while broaching or reaming is performed to establish

Reduction Manouvre

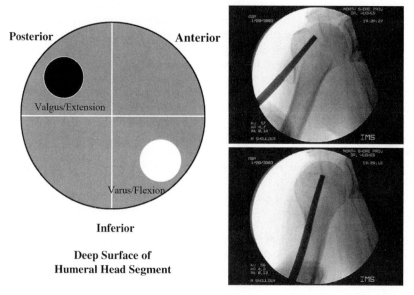

**Deep Surface of
Humeral Head Segment**

Fig. 3. The initial reduction involves correcting the head displacement in relation to the tuberosities. The head segment displacement is often multiplanar. In valgus impacted fractures there is often an extension component. The head segment is elevated by pushing on the posterior/superior surface of the head fracture plane. Varus deformities are reduced by pushing on the anterior/inferior segment. Care should be taken not to disrupt any remaining periosteal medial hinge.

a track for passage of the nail. It is critical to maintain reduction during this phase, controlling rotation with the traction sutures, so that eccentric broaching or reaming does not result in a nail trajectory that displaces the fracture. A guidewire can be used for reaming or insertion of the nail but is often not required in proximal fractures unless comminution extends into the shaft.

Following confirmation of reduction, the nail is inserted to the appropriate depth using manual pressure. The proximal end of the nail must be seated below the articular cartilage and flush with the subchondral bone to prevent impingement against the rotator cuff and this can be checked fluoroscopically. It is important, however, not to countersink the nail more than 5 mm below the subchondral bone because this will place the proximal cross-locking screws in suboptimal positions and also make nail removal difficult. Furthermore, the stability of the construct may be reduced if the proximal nail does not get good purchase in bone, with better-quality bone being in the subchondral region. The proximal cross-locking screws can then be inserted using a targeting guide. Multiple screws are applied at different positions and angles into the tuberosity fragments so that fixation is distributed in the articular segment. Screws are inserted through a cannula

and once the cannula is flush with the bone, the lateral cortex is drilled. It is extremely important to avoid penetration of the articular cartilage of the humeral head while drilling. Not only can this cause direct injury to the glenohumeral joint, it provides a potential pathway for screw migration should the fracture subsequently collapse. It is recommended that a "drill and tap" technique be used for drilling into the humeral head. This technique involves repeatedly pushing the drill without power a short distance as it is advanced through the cancellous bone of the humeral head so as to allow a tactile appreciation of when the harder subchondral bone is reached. Dynamic screening using fluoroscopy is also essential during placement of screws to avoid the complication of screw penetration. Simply obtaining orthogonal views in two planes is not sufficient to exclude screw penetration of the humeral head. Fluoroscopy also confirms that the screw lengths are correct and that the screw heads are flush with the lateral cortex.

If additional fixation of the head complex is required, tension band sutures are generally preferred; however, a combination of screws and sutures or even wires can be used. Muscle forces acting to displace the tuberosity fragments must be counterbalanced. The proximal cross-locking screw heads are used for this purpose, providing a post for suture placement opposite to the individual muscle vectors. The infraspinatus/teres minor tension band suture is secured to the lesser tuberosity cross-locking screw and the subscapularis suture is fixed to the screw located most posterior in the greater tuberosity. Small drill holes are made in the lateral cortex of the proximal shaft to secure the tension band sutures from the supraspinatus, or alternatively a unicortical screw can be used as a post. It is important not to overreduce the tuberosity fragments because this may result in excessive tension in the capsulotendinous structures that may limit motion postoperatively.

In some cases, there is residual shortening of the head complex with relation to the shaft. Fracture healing in this position shortens the lever arm of the deltoid, which may cause problems, including weakness and pain, in some patients. Particularly in young, active individuals, it is important to aim to achieve as near normal function of the shoulder as possible by restoring the native anatomy and biomechanics. To distract the fracture out to length, a laminar spreader can be used laterally abutting the proximal cortex of the shaft and directed against the lower cross-locking screw in the greater tuberosity (Fig. 4). As the laminar spreader is gently opened under fluoroscopic control, a distraction force translates the

shaft distally over the nail until normal length is restored. This position is maintained while static distal cross-locking screws are placed using a targeting device. These cortical screws are inserted percutaneously through an appropriately located small incision. Fluoroscopy is used to confirm correct length of screws and placement through the nail. The shoulder is then taken through a range of motion and fluoroscopy used to make a final assessment of the adequacy of reduction and fracture stability. This final screening should also be used to confirm the absence of any screw penetration into the glenohumeral joint (Fig. 5).

Techniques for managing fracture extension into the shaft and comminution

Proximal humerus fractures can present with extensive comminution, including extension into the proximal third of the shaft. There may be a long medial spike attached to the head fragment or alternatively there may be butterfly fragments located in the medial metadiaphyseal region. These fracture patterns generally result from higher-energy trauma with more extensive injury to the soft tissues and in particular the periosteum. Meticulous surgical technique with careful handling of the soft tissues is especially important in these situations to preserve the vascularity of the humeral head. For stable fixation, a longer

Surgical Neck Fracture
Reduction with Distraction

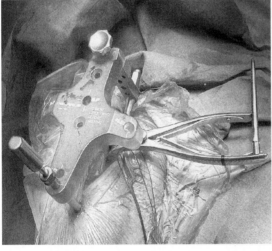 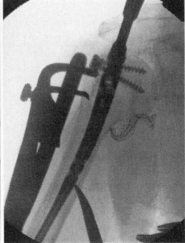

Fig. 4. The tuberosities are fixed to the head and the nail is then introduced in to the canal. The locking screws are directed through the tuberosities. The head/tuberosity segment may require compression or distraction relative to the shaft. The fluoroscopic image depicts a laminar spreader providing distraction.

Proximal Humeral Fracture
Combine Tension Band Suture + Locked Nail

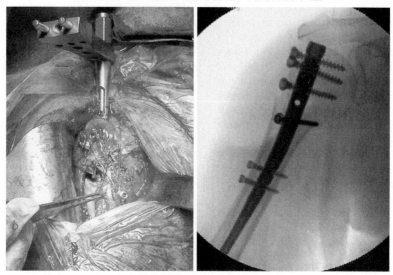

Fig. 5. The rotator cuff segments are then tension-band sutured to the locking screws, which provides improved stability and reduces screw back-out. The distal locking screws are inserted with the correct rotation of the humerus.

nail must be chosen that adequately spans the fracture (eg, Polarus Plus [Acumed, Hillsboro, Oregon, USA]). Additional fixation is provided by proximal cortical cross-locking screws directed into the medial metaphyseal region (Fig. 6) or cerclage wires for widely displaced fragments (taking great care to avoid entrapment of neighboring neurovascular structures). The bicipital groove is often preserved in these cases and is the best guide for assessing rotation during reduction. It is important to remember that proximal cross locking into the head fragment should be performed before any adjustments in the rotation or length of the fracture. Gentle downward traction on the arm may assist in obtaining anatomic fracture reduction through means of ligamentotaxis. This

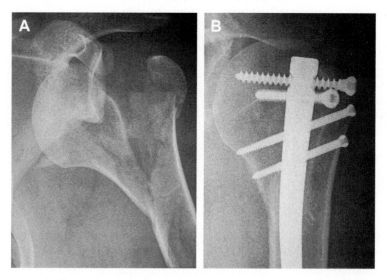

Fig. 6. A patient who had epilepsy presented with a fracture-dislocation of the proximal humerus with a large medial metaphyseal segment (*A*). This was fixated with a locked intramedullary nail and oblique screws (*B*).

practice is recommended mainly in younger patients and care should be taken to avoid overdistraction at the fracture site or disimpacting stably impacted fractures in the elderly, risking possible nonunion. Reaming of the intramedullary canal may be required for the insertion of longer nails, particularly when the canal isthmus is narrow. Gentle reaming to avoid notching is performed over a guidewire and it is recommended to ream to a diameter 1 to 1.5 mm greater than the size of the distal nail to ensure smooth passage of the nail. Radiolucent targeting devices are available for distal cross locking but are often unreliable. Distal cross locking is therefore generally performed using standard "free-hand" fluoroscopic techniques.

Postoperative protocol and rehabilitation

Patients are immobilized postoperatively in 15 degrees of external rotation in an abduction brace to balance the tension in the rotator cuff muscles and neutralize forces acting across the tuberosity fixation. Patients are started on immediate postoperative active elbow and wrist range-of-motion exercises. A passive shoulder range-of-motion exercise program is commenced after 3 weeks when there has been some early healing of the tuberosity fragments. If the lesser tuberosity was intact initially, then external rotation to 30 degrees and forward elevation to 110 degrees is allowed. If repair of the lesser tuberosity was undertaken, then motion is restricted to external rotation to neutral and forward elevation to 90 degrees. Progressive return to full passive range of motion is progressed over the next 3 weeks. At 6 weeks post surgery, patients are commenced on active assisted exercises. Providing the fracture is demonstrating radiographic and clinical evidence of uniting, then strengthening against resistance is allowed at approximately 12 weeks postoperatively.

Results and complications

Locked intramedullary nailing has been used successfully to manage proximal humerus fractures; however, most reports are from retrospective studies involving small series [20–30]. There are no prospective randomized controlled studies published in the literature. We are similarly not aware of any clinical studies currently available in the literature comparing locked intramedullary nailing to other surgical methods of treating proximal humerus fractures. Nonetheless, the results of the limited available studies investigating intramedullary nailing are generally promising with most reporting satisfactory or excellent outcomes in 78% to 89% of patients who had displaced two-, three-, and four-part injuries [23,24,26,28,29]. Mittlmeier and colleagues [25] had complete prospective follow-up data on 50 patients at 1 year following fixation of proximal humerus fractures with locked intramedullary nailing and reported a mean Constant score of 78.8, despite a high complication rate. They found that their results compared favorably with results in the literature following treatment of patients who had minimal osteosynthesis for whom the mean Constant score ranged from 60 to 81 points [19,31–36]. The results of locked intramedullary fixation also compare favorably with recent reported results of fixed-angle plating with mean Constant scores ranging from 62 to 75 points [37–39]. As expected, results following locked intramedullary fixation have not been as good for Neer four-part fractures as they have been for two- and three-part fractures [20,22,25,30]. No difference in functional outcome has been demonstrated between two- and three-part proximal humerus fractures [23,26].

Despite the overall good to excellent results achieved with locked intramedullary fixation of proximal humerus fractures, some studies have reported high rates of complications, up to 50% [21,25,30]. Analysis of the results of available studies reporting on intramedullary nailing of proximal humeral fractures reveals a fairly high overall complication rate of approximately 31% [20–30]. On closer inspection, most of these complications were noted to be minor and easily addressed by the authors. Loosening or backing out of the proximal screws accounted for more than half of the reported complications. Modern implant designs seem to have eliminated this problem and it is therefore expected that future studies should demonstrate significantly lower complication rates [22]. Overall, the occurrence of avascular necrosis following intramedullary nailing is approximately 4.7%, delayed union or nonunion approaching 3%, and stiffness similarly 3%. The rate of avascular necrosis compares favorably to quoted figures in the literature for other methods of internal fixation, including plating techniques with a reported range of 0% to 37% [8,16,37,40–44]. No cases of deep infection have been reported in any of the studies we reviewed using locked intramedullary fixation.

Deep infection complicating fixed-angle plate fixation of proximal humerus fractures has been reported by several authors [37,39,45].

Locked intramedullary fixation of displaced proximal humerus fractures is a technically demanding procedure and should be performed only by experienced surgeons. A recent study by van den Broek and colleagues [30] demonstrated the potential influence of technical aspects of the procedure on the results of intramedullary fixation in displaced two-, three-, and four-part fractures. They reported a high complication rate of 42%, including screw migration, loss of tuberosity reduction (corrected in all cases with revision surgery using additional suture fixation), screw penetration of the glenohumeral joint, and proximal impingement. They also reported malalignment in 9 of 24 patients; most of these were in varus alignment. Almost all of these complications were related to technical failures and therefore should be avoidable. It should be noted that they had no cases of avascular necrosis or nonunion. Others have reported similar complications, including impingement secondary to protrusion of the proximal portion of the nail [24,29,30]. This complication can be avoided by proper seating of the nail below the subchondral bone. Likewise, penetration of the articular cartilage by proximal locking screws has been reported by others [22,29]. Penetration of the articular cartilage of the humeral head is a potentially disastrous complication leading to chondrolysis and early degenerative changes. It is equally important, however, to place screws into the subchondral region of the humeral head to obtain good purchase in better-quality bone. It is therefore imperative to screen intraoperatively with fluoroscopy to achieve optimal proximal locking screw position without risking penetration. Simply obtaining orthogonal views in two planes is not sufficient to exclude screw penetration of the humeral head. It is recommended not to pass through the humeral head articular surface, even when drilling, and to choose screws less than the measured maximum length [22,25].

Agel and colleagues [21] reported on a retrospective series of 20 cases treated with locked intramedullary nailing and noted proximal fixation failure in three patients in whom the fracture pattern extended into the lateral metaphyseal region. They highlighted that nail insertion site is of critical importance in the setting of lateral metaphyseal comminution. Metaphyseal comminution is not an uncommon finding in elderly patients who have osteopenic bone. In addition, difficulty in obtaining secure purchase with locking screws can be anticipated in these situations and it is therefore recommended to augment fixation with tension band sutures. A recent study by Park and colleagues [26] reported results using this technique. They demonstrated no difference in outcome when comparing patients younger than 65 years of age with those older than 65 years of age, suggesting that intramedullary nailing with tension band sutures provides a stable construct in older patients. These results were supported by Rajasekhar and colleagues [28], who actually reported higher functional scores in patients older than 60 years of age.

Summary

Locked intramedullary nailing can be used with success in treating displaced proximal humerus fractures, especially those with complex configurations involving the head, metaphysis, and shaft. It is a technically demanding procedure, however, with a potentially high complication rate.

References

[1] Stableforth PG. Four-part fractures of the neck of the humerus. J Bone Joint Surg Br 1984;66(1):104–8.

[2] Misra A, Kapur R, Maffulli N. Complex proximal humeral fractures in adults—a systematic review of management. Injury 2001;32(5):363–72.

[3] Handoll HH, Gibson JN, Madhok R. Interventions for treating proximal humeral fractures in adults. Cochrane Database Syst Rev 2003;(4):CD000434.

[4] Bong MR, Kummer FJ, Koval KJ, et al. Intramedullary nailing of the lower extremity: biomechanics and biology. J Am Acad Orthop Surg 2007;15(2):97–106.

[5] Hessmann MH, Hansen WS, Krummenauer F, et al. Locked plate fixation and intramedullary nailing for proximal humerus fractures: a biomechanical evaluation. J Trauma 2005;58(6):1194–201.

[6] Kitson J, Booth G, Day R. A biomechanical comparison of locking plate and locking nail implants used for fractures of the proximal humerus. J Shoulder Elbow Surg 2007;16(3):362–6.

[7] Fuchtmeier B, May R, Hente R, et al. Proximal humerus fractures: a comparative biomechanical analysis of intra and extramedullary implants. Arch Orthop Trauma Surg 2007;127(6):441–7.

[8] Gerber C, Werner CM, Vienne P. Internal fixation of complex fractures of the proximal humerus. J Bone Joint Surg Br 2004;86(6):848–55.

[9] Neer CS 2nd. Displaced proximal humeral fractures. II. Treatment of three-part and four-part displacement. J Bone Joint Surg Am 1970;52(6):1090–103.

[10] Hertel R, Hempfing A, Stiehler M, et al. Predictors of humeral head ischemia after intracapsular fracture of the proximal humerus. J Shoulder Elbow Surg 2004;13(4):427–33.

[11] Mighell MA, Kolm GP, Collinge CA, et al. Outcomes of hemiarthroplasty for fractures of the proximal humerus. J Shoulder Elbow Surg 2003; 12(6):569–77.

[12] Robinson CM, Khan LA, Akhtar MA. Treatment of anterior fracture-dislocations of the proximal humerus by open reduction and internal fixation. J Bone Joint Surg Br 2006;88(4):502–8.

[13] Robinson CM, Page RS, Hill RM, et al. Primary hemiarthroplasty for treatment of proximal humeral fractures. J Bone Joint Surg Am 2003;85(7):1215–23.

[14] Kralinger F, Schwaiger R, Wambacher M, et al. Outcome after primary hemiarthroplasty for fracture of the head of the humerus. A retrospective multicentre study of 167 patients. J Bone Joint Surg Br 2004;86(2):217–9.

[15] Gerber C, Hersche O, Berberat C. The clinical relevance of posttraumatic avascular necrosis of the humeral head. J Shoulder Elbow Surg 1998;7(6): 586–90.

[16] Wijgman AJ, Roolker W, Patt TW, et al. Open reduction and internal fixation of three and four-part fractures of the proximal part of the humerus. J Bone Joint Surg Am. 2002;84(11):1919–25.

[17] Iannotti JP, Ramsey ML, Williams GR Jr, et al. Nonprosthetic management of proximal humeral fractures. Instr Course Lect 2004;53:403–16.

[18] Nho SJ, Brophy RH, Barker JU, et al. Innovations in the management of displaced proximal humerus fractures. J Am Acad Orthop Surg 2007;15(1):12–26.

[19] Resch H, Beck E, Bayley I. Reconstruction of the valgus-impacted humeral head fracture. J Shoulder Elbow Surg 1995;4(2):73–80.

[20] Adedapo AO, Ikpeme JO. The results of internal fixation of three- and four-part proximal humeral fractures with the Polarus nail. Injury 2001;32(2): 115–21.

[21] Agel J, Jones CB, Sanzone AG, et al. Treatment of proximal humeral fractures with Polarus nail fixation. J Shoulder Elbow Surg 2004;13(2):191–5.

[22] Gradl G, Dietze A, Arndt D, et al. Angular and sliding stable antegrade nailing (Targon PH) for the treatment of proximal humeral fractures. Arch Orthop Trauma Surg 2007;127(10):937–44.

[23] Kazakos K, Lyras DN, Galanis V, et al. Internal fixation of proximal humerus fractures using the Polarus intramedullary nail. Arch Orthop Trauma Surg 2007;127(7):503–8.

[24] Lin J, Hou SM, Hang YS. Locked nailing for displaced surgical neck fractures of the humerus. J Trauma 1998;45(6):1051–7.

[25] Mittlmeier TW, Stedtfeld HW, Ewert A, et al. Stabilization of proximal humeral fractures with an angular and sliding stable antegrade locking nail (Targon PH). J Bone Joint Surg Am 2003; 85(Suppl 4):136–46.

[26] Park JY, An JW, Oh JH. Open intramedullary nailing with tension band and locking sutures for proximal humeral fracture: hot air balloon technique. J Shoulder Elbow Surg 2006;15(5):594–601.

[27] Parsons M, O'Brien J, Hughes J. Locked intramedullary nailing for displaced and unstable proximal humerus fractures. Techn Shoulder Elbow Surg 2005;6(2):75–86.

[28] Rajasekhar C, Ray PS, Bhamra MS. Fixation of proximal humeral fractures with the Polarus nail. J Shoulder Elbow Surg 2001;10(1):7–10.

[29] Sosef N, Stobbe I, Hogervorst M, et al. The Polarus intramedullary nail for proximal humeral fractures: outcome in 28 patients followed for 1 year. Acta Orthop 2007;78(3):436–41.

[30] van den Broek CM, van den Besselaar M, Coenen JM, et al. Displaced proximal humeral fractures: intramedullary nailing versus conservative treatment. Arch Orthop Trauma Surg 2007;127(6): 459–63.

[31] Ko JY, Yamamoto R. Surgical treatment of complex fracture of the proximal humerus. Clin Orthop Relat Res 1996;327:225–37.

[32] Resch H, Povacz P, Frohlich R, et al. Percutaneous fixation of three- and four-part fractures of the proximal humerus. J Bone Joint Surg Br 1997; 79(2):295–300.

[33] Resch H, Hubner C, Schwaiger R. Minimally invasive reduction and osteosynthesis of articular fractures of the humeral head. Injury 2001;32(Suppl 1): SA25–32.

[34] Schai P, Imhoff A, Preiss S. Comminuted humeral head fractures: a multicenter analysis. J Shoulder Elbow Surg 1995;4(5):319–30.

[35] Zyto K, Ahrengart L, Sperber A, et al. Treatment of displaced proximal humeral fractures in elderly patients. J Bone Joint Surg Br 1997;79(3):412–7.

[36] Zyto K, Kronberg M, Brostrom LA. Shoulder function after displaced fractures of the proximal humerus. J Shoulder Elbow Surg 1995;4(5):331–6.

[37] Fankhauser F, Boldin C, Schippinger G, et al. A new locking plate for unstable fractures of the proximal humerus. Clin Orthop Relat Res 2005;430:176–81.

[38] Lill H, Hepp P, Rose T, et al. [The angle stable locking-proximal-humerus-plate (LPHP) for proximal humeral fractures using a small anterior-lateral-deltoid-splitting-approach—technique and first results]. Zentralbl Chir 2004;129(1):43–8 [in German].

[39] Plecko M, Kraus A. Internal fixation of proximal humerus fractures using the locking proximal humerus plate. Oper Orthop Traumatol 2005; 17(1):25–50.

[40] Esser RD. Open reduction and internal fixation of three- and four-part fractures of the proximal humerus. Clin Orthop Relat Res 1994;(299): 244–51.

[41] Hintermann B, Trouillier HH, Schafer D. Rigid internal fixation of fractures of the proximal humerus in older patients. J Bone Joint Surg Br 2000;82(8): 1107–12.

[42] Hawkins RJ, Bell RH, Gurr K. The three-part fracture of the proximal part of the humerus. Operative treatment. J Bone Joint Surg Am 1986;68(9): 1410–4.

[43] Sturzenegger M, Fornaro E, Jakob RP. Results of surgical treatment of multifragmented fractures of the humeral head. Arch Orthop Trauma Surg 1982;100(4):249–59.

[44] Hente R, Kampshoff J, Kinner B, et al. [Treatment of dislocated 3- and 4-part fractures of the proximal humerus with an angle-stabilizing fixation plate]. Unfallchirurg 2004;107(9):769–82 [in German].

[45] Voigt C, Woltmann A, Partenheimer A, et al. [Management of complications after angularly stable locking proximal humerus plate fixation]. Chirurg 2007;78(1):40–6 [in German].

ELSEVIER
SAUNDERS

Orthop Clin N Am 39 (2008) 429–439

ORTHOPEDIC
CLINICS
OF NORTH AMERICA

Open Reduction and Internal Fixation of Proximal Humerus Fractures

Darren S. Drosdowech, MD, FRCSC[a,b,*],
Kenneth J. Faber, MD, MHPE, FRCSC[a,b],
George S. Athwal, MD, FRCSC[a,b]

[a]Hand and Upper Limb Centre, St. Joseph's Health Care, University of Western Ontario,
268 Grosvenor Street, London, Ontario, Canada N6A 4V2
[b]Department of Surgery, University of Western Ontario, London, Ontario, Canada N6A 3K7

Fractures of the proximal humerus are common and can have a profound effect on the quality of life of patients. Kannus and colleagues [1] reported an incidence of 40 proximal humerus fractures per 100,000 patients older than 60 years of age. They also projected a threefold increase in the incidence of this injury over the next 30 years. Court-Brown and colleagues [2] have stated that "proximal humerus fractures often occur in the fit elderly independent patient who is still a net contributor to society but who might well be converted to a degree of social dependency by the fracture."

Evidence-based recommendations to guide treatment of this injury are lacking. A recent systematic review [3] and a Cochrane Review on the outcomes of surgical treatment of proximal humeral fractures made several interesting findings [4]. The authors found that no good evidence exists whether surgery is clearly superior to nonoperative treatment. When surgery was performed, the available data were inconclusive in identifying what type of procedure was most effective for a particular fracture pattern. The authors concluded that although numerous publications exist describing various techniques in the management of proximal humerus fractures, the development of evidence-based treatment guidelines was challenging. This article outlines the technical aspects, outcomes, and complications of open reduction and internal fixation of proximal humeral fractures.

Classification

Numerous classification systems for proximal humeral fractures have been described. An extension of Codman's [5] observations, Neer [6] introduced the concept of "parts" based on the epiphyseal growth centers that collectively compose the proximal humerus. Although steeped in tradition and arguably a standard language used by most orthopedic surgeons, the inter- and intra-observer reliability of Neer's classification system is low [7–9]. The AO classification originally described by Müller has also been used but has similar limitations in reliability [7] and prognosis [9,10].

Recently, Hertel and colleagues [11] described a proximal humerus fracture classification scheme that included an anatomic description of the fracture based on 12 possible configurations and outlined factors that predicted the likelihood of humeral head ischemia. Factors associated with humeral head ischemia include disruption of the medial periosteal hinge, medial metadiaphyseal extension of less than 8 mm, increasing fracture complexity, and displacement of greater than 10 mm or angulation greater than 45 degrees. Although Hertel's classification method improves our understanding of injury patterns and aids in surgical decision making, it does not indicate which fractures are best treated with operative management versus nonoperative management.

* Corresponding author.
  E-mail address: ddros@mac.com (D.S. Drosdowech).

Interpretation of imaging remains the cornerstone of assessing fracture geometry. Standard radiographs include anteroposterior, lateral scapular, and axillary views. Additional information can be obtained with two- or three-dimensional CT scanning; however, this imaging modality is also subject to significant inter- and intraobserver variability [12–14]. A combination of imaging studies is often necessary to provide a clear understanding of the fracture pattern, displacement, and angulation before deciding on treatment.

Decision making

The decision to operate on a particular fracture relies on several factors, including fracture pattern/classification, the natural history of the fracture, patient-related factors, and surgeon-related factors. Patient factors include age, bone quality, status of the rotator cuff, hand dominance, smoking status, the presence of pre-existing joint pathology, medical comorbidities, and anticipated postoperative compliance. Surgeon-related issues include selection of a particular fixation device or technique, recognition and treatment of associated injuries (ie, glenoid fracture, acute rotator cuff tear), timing of surgery, and appropriate direction of postoperative rehabilitation. A fracture that would typically be amenable to open surgical repair may be treated nonsurgically when additional patient or surgeon-related cofactors are evident.

Although the focus of this article is on open reduction and internal fixation of proximal humerus fractures, other treatment modalities should always be considered. Several authors have demonstrated high rates of patient satisfaction with nonsurgical treatment of displaced and angulated proximal humerus fractures, despite residual malunion [15–17]. Fjalestad and colleagues [18] concluded that surgery did not benefit their patients who had complex, displaced fractures when compared with a cohort of patients managed nonoperatively.

Anatomic neck fractures

Fractures of the anatomic humeral head neck junction are exceedingly rare. When these fractures occur in the elderly, humeral hemiarthroplasty is indicated given the high incidence of posttraumatic avascular necrosis of the humeral head. In younger patients, open reduction and internal fixation is certainly indicated despite the risk for avascular necrosis, leaving arthroplasty as a late reconstructive option if necessary.

The fractures are typically approached through the deltopectoral interval. Stable internal fixation of the humeral head can be challenging because of its small size combined with the difficult exposure encountered with an intact rotator cuff and tuberosities. Achieving the necessary surgical exposure is a balance, because further exposure risks damage to the vital blood supply of the humeral head. The arcuate branch of the anterior circumflex humeral artery ascends in the bicipital groove lateral to the long head of the biceps and is at risk for injury during surgical dissection [19–22]. Opening the rotator interval tissue may assist in reducing the humeral head but may not permit enough exposure for stable internal fixation, such as the insertion of headless compression screws. A combination of antegrade and retrograde fixation may be the best method of fixation in these unique circumstances.

Surgical neck fractures (with or without tuberosity involvement)

Displaced fractures of the surgical neck of the humerus are often managed by open reduction and internal fixation. Open reduction allows for direct control of individual fracture fragments and permits the application of rigid fixation. Numerous methods have been used to achieve these goals and have ranged from intramedullary devices, tension band or cerclage sutures/wires, plates, or a combination of these methods.

Techniques for internal fixation of proximal humerus fractures continue to evolve. Despite the popularity of proximal humerus locking plates it is important to recognize that other reasonable alternatives were often used not long ago, and still may be valid treatment options. Transosseous suture fixation [23] has been shown to be an effective fixation technique, although Williams and colleagues [24] have shown that intramedullary devices when combined with a tension band construct provide more rigid fixation than tension banding alone. Disadvantages of this technique include the need to violate the supraspinatus tendon insertion to allow passage of the intramedullary device and the difficulties that can be encountered if the hardware requires removal. The addition of bone graft or a bone graft substitute may be necessary in nonunions of the surgical neck, but are rarely needed in acute fractures. Some degree of shortening of the humerus is well tolerated by impacting the shaft into the wider metaphyseal segment to achieve further fracture stability and avoiding the use of bone graft.

Plates have been used to achieve more rigid fixation of surgical neck fractures permitting earlier postoperative range of motion. Large fragment plates, such as the AO T-plate [25] or cloverleaf plate [26], have been used most often and generally require contouring to fit the proximal humerus. Plate application should not violate the attachments of the rotator cuff. Plate/screw constructs have the greatest stability when screws are directed toward the center of the humeral head and positioned just beneath the subchondral bone [27]. The disadvantages of plate fixation include the risk for damaging the blood supply to the humeral head during dissection and failure of the fixation construct with screw migration in weak osteopenic bone.

The introduction of fixed-angle devices to the proximal humerus resolved some of the problems associated with poor purchase in osteopenic bone. Blade plates [28] are commercially available or they can be made intraoperatively by bending conventional plates [29]. Although blade plates are more structurally rigid than conventional plates, their disadvantages include their higher profile, which at times causes impingement necessitating removal, and their limited proximal screw options.

The advent of locking plate technology revolutionized fixation in osteopenic bone. Fracture-specific implants, such as precontoured proximal humerus locking plates that conform to the anatomy of the proximal humerus, are now commercially available (Fig. 1). These devices allow the placement of convergent and divergent locking screws that permit multiple points of fixation within osteopenic bone creating a fixed-angle device that captures a volume of bone. Seide and colleagues [30] compare locked to unlocked plating constructs in the proximal humerus and demonstrated a 74% higher static stiffness and significantly more cycles to failure under dynamic loads in the locked screw construct. Most precontoured proximal humerus locking plates have other fracture-specific adaptations, such as peripheral holes for provisional Kirschner-wire fixation or for suture fixation of individual tuberosity or bone fragments. The reported early clinical results with the precontoured proximal humerus locking plates have been favorable [31,32].

Authors' preferred technique

The patient is positioned semisitting (beach-chair) on a specialized operating room table (T-max, Tenet Calgary, AB, Canada) that allows access to the shoulder and unimpeded intraoperative fluoroscopy. The C-arm unit is brought in from the opposite side of the patient to avoid interfering with the surgical team's access to the operative site. Fluoroscopy is done preoperatively, before sterile prep and drape, to ensure the required images are attainable (Fig. 2).

An anterior shoulder skin incision is used, while the deep approach uses the deltopectoral

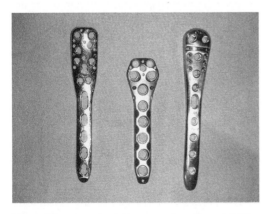

Fig. 1. Three representative examples of proximal humeral locking plates (left to right: Synthes 3.5-mm LCP, Zimmer NCB plate, Aequalis humeral plate).

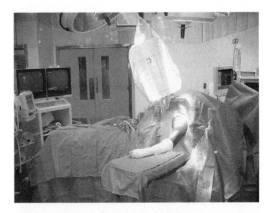

Fig. 2. Intraoperative setup during open reduction and internal fixation of a proximal humeral fracture. Note the C-arm coming in on the opposite side of the operative shoulder.

interval. If the procedure is done early (within 3–5 days) the ability to identify individual fracture fragments is technically easier. The intact long head of biceps tendon can be used to as a guide to the intertubercular groove and therefore the tuberosities and rotator cuff interval. If the biceps tendon has been lacerated because of sharp fracture fragments, the intertubercular groove can be used as a landmark. Excessive dissection around the groove is avoided to minimize the possibility of further devascularization of the humeral head. The axillary nerve should be palpated anterior to the subscapularis muscle and posteriorly as it exits the quadrilateral space to innervate the deltoid and teres minor muscles.

Release of the subdeltoid, subacromial and subcoracoid recesses improves visualization and mobilization of the fracture fragments. If the proximal fragments are osteopenic and difficult to control with standard reduction techniques (ie, reduction forceps), provisional sutures (#1 braided absorbable) may be used at the cuff/tuberosity junction to help control the fragments during reduction. If the lesser or greater tuberosity fragments are also involved they can be individually sutured at the tendon-bone junction and later incorporated into the fixed construct using #2 braided high-density sutures through the locking plate's small peripheral holes (Fig. 3). Careful mobilization and elevation of an impacted head fragment often leaves a metaphyseal bone defect that may require bone graft or graft substitute. The graft material should be placed beneath the humeral head and deep to the tuberosities to assist the locking plate in maintaining reduction (Fig. 4).

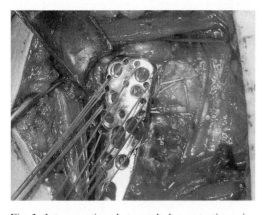

Fig. 3. Intraoperative photograph demonstrating using the peripheral holes in the locking plate for greater and lesser tuberosity suture fixation.

The locking plate is applied to the anterolateral proximal humerus just posterior to the bicipital groove, approximately 0.5 to 1 cm below the tip of the greater tuberosity to limit postoperative subacromial plate impingement. Release of the anterior third of the deltoid insertion may be required to appropriately position the distal aspect of the plate on the humeral shaft. Screws placed through the plate are used to fixate the head to the shaft and when necessary the greater tuberosity to the head and shaft. The lesser tuberosity usually cannot be fixated with screws placed through the locking plate and therefore usually requires suture fixation. It has been shown that placement of locking screws into the inferomedial aspect of the humeral head improves fracture stability (Fig. 5) [33]. The goal of open reduction and internal fixation is to obtain anatomic reduction of all the bony fragments with rigid fixation to allow early range of motion.

Isolated greater tuberosity fractures

Displaced, isolated fractures of the greater tuberosity usually require surgical reduction and internal fixation. These fractures can occur in conjunction with traumatic anterior shoulder dislocations and associated pathology may be present that requires treatment (glenoid fractures, subscapularis tendon tears). In addition to standard shoulder radiographs, an anteroposterior radiograph with the shoulder in external rotation has demonstrated improved accuracy in diagnosing minimally displaced (≤ 5 mm) fractures [34].

The degree of displacement necessitating fracture reduction remains unanswered. Traditionally, greater tuberosity displacement 10 mm or greater has been suggested as a surgical indication, because favorable outcomes have been demonstrated in the literature [35]. Platzer and colleagues [36], however, suggested that lesser degrees of displacement may benefit from surgical reduction and fixation. Bono and colleagues [37] have shown that the force required to abduct the arm in a cadaveric model significantly increases with superior greater tuberosity displacement as little as 5 mm.

Authors' preferred technique

The patient is positioned in the beach-chair fashion with C-arm fluoroscopy available. Reduction and fixation are accomplished through a deltoid splitting approach located along the

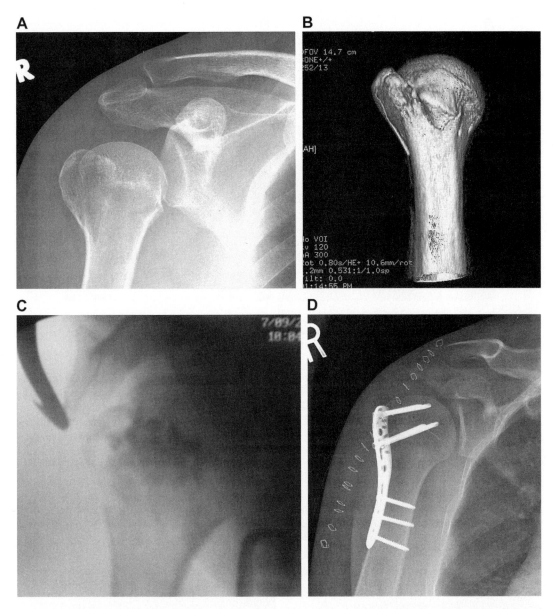

Fig. 4. Preoperative anteroposterior radiograph (*A*) and three-dimensional CT image demonstrating a valgus impacted proximal humerus fracture in a young active 40-year-old man. (*B*) Intraoperative fluoroscopy (*C*) demonstrating metaphyseal grafting with additional plate fixation to elevate the head into anatomic position (*D*).

tendinous raphe between the anterior and middle thirds of the deltoid. By varying the degree of humeral rotation, the anterior and posterior aspects of the tuberosity fracture fragments can be accessed as can any associated tendon or rotator interval injuries.

The size and bone quality of the tuberosity fragment determines the type of fixation used.

Larger fragments with good bone quality permit the use of screw fixation with multiple partially threaded compression screws with or without washers (Fig. 6). The screws should be placed below the tip of the greater tuberosity to prevent impingement in abduction or forward elevation. Large fragments can also be fixed rigidly with locking plates (Fig. 7). Smaller tuberosity

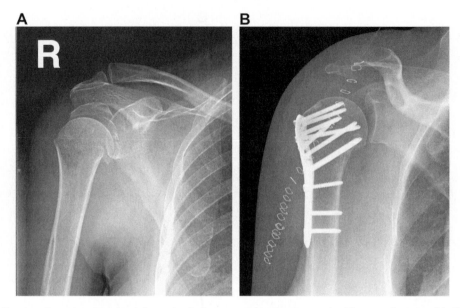

Fig. 5. Preoperative anteroposterior radiograph of a four-part valgus impact proximal humerus fracture with disruption of the medial periosteal hinge (*A*). The fracture underwent open reduction and locked plate fixation with screws directed into the inferomedial portion of the humeral head to provide maximum stability (*B*).

fragments with poor bone quality that do not allow internal fixation with screws are best treated as large rotator cuff tears with a combination of suture anchors or tension band sutures (Fig. 8). To improve stability, the rotator interval may also be suture repaired.

Isolated lesser tuberosity fractures

Isolated fractures of the lesser tuberosity are rare. This injury is often overlooked; therefore, many are treated late. Computed tomography or axillary lateral radiographs may be used to confirm the diagnosis [38]. Late clinical presentation can be deceptive and may reveal restricted internal rotation and subscapularis weakness. This injury, although rare, has a higher prevalence in adolescents. This prevalence is theorized to occur because of a weak zone in the closing physeal growth plate (Fig. 9) [39].

The surgical indications for lesser tuberosity fractures are variably reported in the literature

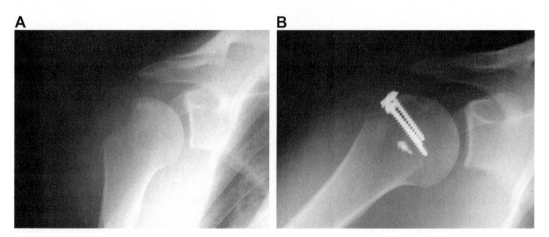

Fig. 6. Preoperative (*A*) and postoperative (*B*) radiographs of an isolated greater tuberosity fracture fixed with multiple screws. The fragment was large with good bone quality.

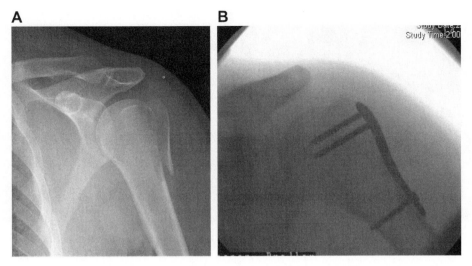

Fig. 7. A large greater tuberosity fracture (*A*) treated with open reduction and internal fixation by way of a percutaneous approach (*B*).

and no consensus has been established [38–40]. In general, anatomic reduction and stable internal fixation can be justified in most displaced fractures because the subscapularis is an important contributor to overall shoulder function [41]. Early intervention may also be preferred because chronic deficiency of this tendon is difficult to manage successfully [42–44].

Authors' preferred technique

The lesser tuberosity fracture is exposed through the deltopectoral interval. The fracture fragment is often retracted inferomedially because of the action of the subscapularis muscle. Subluxation or dislocation of the long head of biceps tendon is often an associated finding and tenotomy or tenodesis is recommended. The fracture surface on the humerus may be obscured by fibrous tissue and should be conservatively débrided, avoiding removing useful humeral metaphyseal bone. In some chronic cases, the lesser tuberosity fragment may be a small cortical shell. In these cases, if the bone is poor quality, the remaining bone fragments can be excised and the tendon repaired directly to bone. When mobilizing the retracted subscapularis tendon, care should be taken to protect adjacent neurovascular

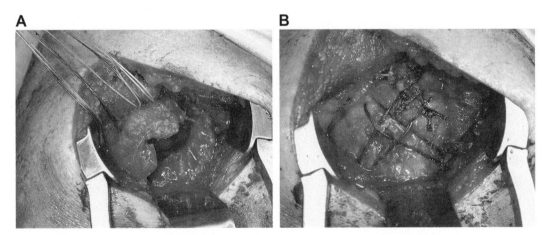

Fig. 8. Intraoperative photographs of greater tuberosity fixation achieved using a combination of suture anchors (*A*) and tension band suture (*B*) technique.

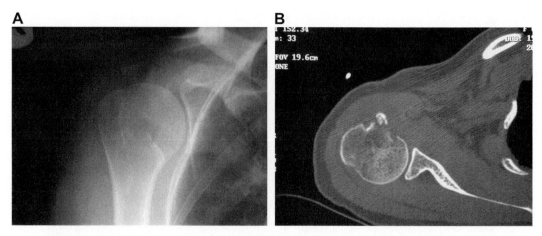

Fig. 9. Anteroposterior radiograph (A) with cross-sectional CT cut (B) demonstrating an isolated lesser tuberosity fracture.

structures, such as the axillary nerve, musculocutaneous nerve, and the axillary and anterior circumflex vessels. If the lesser tuberosity fragment is of sufficient size and quality, it may be fixated with lag screws or a small plate. Tuberosity fixation can also be accomplished with sutures, with suture anchors placed along the anatomic neck to secure the medial aspect of the fragment and with transosseous sutures securing the lateral aspect through bone tunnels placed in the floor of the bicipital groove (Fig. 10).

Stable internal fixation allows for early active-assisted range of motion that may facilitate postoperative rehabilitation. In cases of tenuous fixation, rehabilitation may be delayed to maximize bone healing.

Complications

A thorough discussion of complications associated with the treatment of proximal humeral fractures is beyond the scope of this article. A few complications merit special consideration, however.

Despite their several advantages, proximal humerus locking plates have experienced some failures. Tolat and colleagues [45] reported a case of fatigue failure with the titanium Philos plate (Synthes, Davos, Switzerland). This mechanical failure was attributable to the relatively thin contour of the plate, the notch sensitivity of titanium, and the bending moments experienced by the plate because of the lack of medial calcar support. We have had similar mechanical failures of the stainless

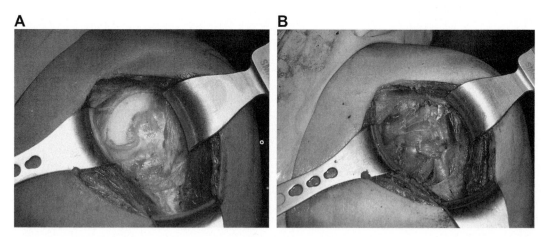

Fig. 10. Pre- (A) and postfixation (B) intraoperative photos of open reduction and internal fixation of a lesser tuberosity fracture in a young patient.

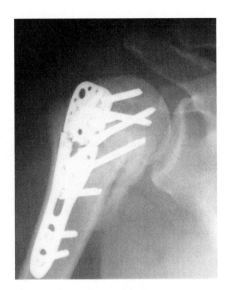

Fig. 11. Complication of a fractured proximal humeral locking plate associated with nonunion of the fracture.

steel model of this plate in cases of delayed union (Fig. 11). Cantilever bending moments that may be the cause of fatigue failure of these plates can be minimized by ensuring medial calcar support, filling the vulnerable screw holes, or by using a thicker plate with similar design features.

Humeral head avascular necrosis is certainly a common complication after displaced multifragment fractures of the proximal humerus. Gerber and colleagues [46] have noted that the functional results after avascular necrosis can be acceptable despite humeral head collapse, as long as the principles of anatomic reduction of the proximal humeral fragments have been respected. In cases of symptomatic head collapse requiring revision to a humeral hemiarthroplasty, the outcomes are superior when the tuberosities have anatomically healed versus those with malunion.

Surgeons should also be cautious when placing the most proximal locking screws into subchondral humeral epiphyseal bone while using modern fixed-angle locking plates. Careful interpretation of intraoperative fluoroscopic imaging throughout a full range of passive motion while placing subchondral head screws should help to reduce the incidence of inadvertent joint penetration and subsequent unwanted iatrogenic chondral injury.

Summary

Open reduction of proximal humeral fractures has the advantage of providing direct control over each fracture fragment and permitting anatomic reduction and fixation with advanced devices. Modern fixed-angle locking plates designed specifically for proximal humerus fractures have allowed the expansion of surgical indications permitting surgeons to address more complicated fractures. Advanced preoperative imaging and fluoroscopy allow a better understanding of fracture patterns and permit the surgeon to use this knowledge intraoperatively. Research is required to further validate fracture classification systems, to develop surgical guidelines for decision making, and to compare the outcomes of the various treatments options for proximal humerus fractures.

References

[1] Kannus P, Palvanen M, Niemi S, et al. Osteoporotic fractures of the proximal humerus in elderly Finnish persons: sharp increase in 1970–1998 and alarming projections for the new millennium. Acta Orthop Scand 2000;71(5):465–70.

[2] Court-Brown CM, Garg A, McQueen MM. The epidemiology of proximal humeral fractures. Acta Orthop Scand 2001;72(4):365–71.

[3] Lanting B, MacDermid J, Drosdowech DS, et al. Proximal humeral fractures: a systematic review of treatment modalities. J Shoulder Elbow Surg 2008; 17(1):42–54.

[4] Gibson JN, Handoll HH, Madhok R. Interventions for treating proximal humeral fractures in adults. Cochrane Database Syst Rev 2001;(1):CD000434.

[5] Codman E. The shoulder, rupture of the supraspinatus tendon and other lesions in or about the subacromial bursa, vol. 2nd edition. Boston: Thomas Todd; 1984.

[6] Neer CS 2nd. Displaced proximal humeral fractures. I. Classification and evaluation. J Bone Joint Surg Am 1970;52(6):1077–89.

[7] Brien H, Noftall F, MacMaster S, et al. Neer's classification system: a critical appraisal. J Trauma 1995; 38(2):257–60.

[8] Sidor ML, Zuckerman JD, Lyon T, et al. The Neer classification system for proximal humeral fractures. An assessment of interobserver reliability and intraobserver reproducibility. J Bone Joint Surg Am 1993;75(12):1745–50.

[9] Siebenrock KA, Gerber C. The reproducibility of classification of fractures of the proximal end of the humerus. J Bone Joint Surg Am 1993;75(12): 1751–5.

[10] Muller M, Nazarian S, Koch P. The comprehensive classification of fractures of long bones. Berlin: Springer Verlag; 1990.

[11] Hertel R, Hempfing A, Stiehler M, et al. Predictors of humeral head ischemia after intracapsular

fracture of the proximal humerus. J Shoulder Elbow Surg 2004;13(4):427–33.

[12] Bernstein J, Adler LM, Blank JE, et al. Evaluation of the Neer system of classification of proximal humeral fractures with computerized tomographic scans and plain radiographs. J Bone Joint Surg Am 1996;78(9):1371–5.

[13] Sjoden GO, Movin T, Aspelin P, et al. 3D-radiographic analysis does not improve the Neer and AO classifications of proximal humeral fractures. Acta Orthop Scand 1999;70(4):325–8.

[14] Sjoden GO, Movin T, Guntner P, et al. Poor reproducibility of classification of proximal humeral fractures. Additional CT of minor value. Acta Orthop Scand 1997;68(3):239–42.

[15] Zyto K, Kronberg M, Brostrom LA. Shoulder function after displaced fractures of the proximal humerus. J Shoulder Elbow Surg 1995;4(5):331–6.

[16] Court-Brown CM, McQueen MM. The impacted varus (A2.2) proximal humeral fracture: prediction of outcome and results of nonoperative treatment in 99 patients. Acta Orthop Scand 2004;75(6):736–40.

[17] Court-Brown CM, Cattermole H, McQueen MM. Impacted valgus fractures (B1.1) of the proximal humerus. The results of non-operative treatment. J Bone Joint Surg Br 2002;84(4):504–8.

[18] Fjalestad T, Stromsoe K, Blucher J, et al. Fractures in the proximal humerus: functional outcome and evaluation of 70 patients treated in hospital. Arch Orthop Trauma Surg 2005;125(5):310–6.

[19] Brooks CH, Revell WJ, Heatley FW. Vascularity of the humeral head after proximal humeral fractures. An anatomical cadaver study. J Bone Joint Surg Br 1993;75(1):132–6.

[20] Duparc F, Muller JM, Freger P. Arterial blood supply of the proximal humeral epiphysis. Surg Radiol Anat 2001;23(3):185–90.

[21] Gerber C, Schneeberger AG, Vinh TS. The arterial vascularization of the humeral head. An anatomical study. J Bone Joint Surg Am 1990;72(10):1486–94.

[22] Meyer C, Alt V, Hassanin H, et al. The arteries of the humeral head and their relevance in fracture treatment. Surg Radiol Anat 2005;27(3):232–7.

[23] Dimakopoulos P, Panagopoulos A, Kasimatis G, et al. Anterior traumatic shoulder dislocation associated with displaced greater tuberosity fracture: the necessity of operative treatment. J Orthop Trauma 2007;21(2):104–12.

[24] Williams GR Jr, Copley LA, Iannotti JP, et al. The influence of intramedullary fixation on figure-of-eight wiring for surgical neck fractures of the proximal humerus: a biomechanical comparison. J Shoulder Elbow Surg 1997;6(5):423–8.

[25] Wijgman AJ, Roolker W, Patt TW, et al. Open reduction and internal fixation of three and four-part fractures of the proximal part of the humerus. J Bone Joint Surg Am 2002;84-A(11):1919–25.

[26] Robinson CM, Page RS. Severely impacted valgus proximal humeral fractures. J Bone Joint Surg Am 2004;86-A(Suppl 1 Pt 2):143–55.

[27] Liew AS, Johnson JA, Patterson SD, et al. Effect of screw placement on fixation in the humeral head. J Shoulder Elbow Surg 2000;9(5):423–6.

[28] Synthes. 4.5 mm cannulated humeral blade plate. Product monograph. Paoli (PA): Synthes; 1998.

[29] Instrum K, Fennell C, Shrive N, et al. Semitubular blade plate fixation in proximal humeral fractures: a biomechanical study in a cadaveric model. J Shoulder Elbow Surg 1998;7(5):462–6.

[30] Seide K, Triebe J, Faschingbauer M, et al. Locked vs. unlocked plate osteosynthesis of the proximal humerus—a biomechanical study. Clin Biomech (Bristol, Avon) 2007;22(2):176–82.

[31] Rose PS, Adams CR, Torchia ME, et al. Locking plate fixation for proximal humeral fractures: initial results with a new implant. J Shoulder Elbow Surg 2007;16(2):202–7.

[32] Fankhauser F, Boldin C, Schippinger G, et al. A new locking plate for unstable fractures of the proximal humerus. Clin Orthop Relat Res 2005;430:176–81.

[33] Gardner MJ, Weil Y, Barker JU, et al. The importance of medial support in locked plating of proximal humerus fractures. J Orthop Trauma 2007;21(3):185–91.

[34] Parsons BO, Klepps SJ, Miller S, et al. Reliability and reproducibility of radiographs of greater tuberosity displacement. A cadaveric study. J Bone Joint Surg Am 2005;87(1):58–65.

[35] Flatow EL, Cuomo F, Maday MG, et al. Open reduction and internal fixation of two-part displaced fractures of the greater tuberosity of the proximal part of the humerus. J Bone Joint Surg Am 1991;73(8):1213–8.

[36] Platzer P, Kutscha-Lissberg F, Lehr S, et al. The influence of displacement on shoulder function in patients with minimally displaced fractures of the greater tuberosity. Injury 2005;36(10):1185–9.

[37] Bono CM, Renard R, Levine RG, et al. Effect of displacement of fractures of the greater tuberosity on the mechanics of the shoulder. J Bone Joint Surg Br 2001;83(7):1056–62.

[38] van Laarhoven HA, te Slaa RL, van Laarhoven EW. Isolated avulsion fracture of the lesser tuberosity of the humerus. J Trauma 1995;39(5):997–9.

[39] Levine B, Pereira D, Rosen J. Avulsion fractures of the lesser tuberosity of the humerus in adolescents: review of the literature and case report. J Orthop Trauma 2005;19(5):349–52.

[40] Ogawa K, Takahashi M. Long-term outcome of isolated lesser tuberosity fractures of the humerus. J Trauma 1997;42(5):955–9.

[41] Kelly BT, Williams RJ, Cordasco FA, et al. Differential patterns of muscle activation in patients with symptomatic and asymptomatic rotator cuff tears. J Shoulder Elbow Surg 2005;14(2):165–71.

[42] Jost B, Puskas GJ, Lustenberger A, et al. Outcome of pectoralis major transfer for the treatment of irreparable subscapularis tears. J Bone Joint Surg Am 2003;85-A(10):1944–51.

[43] Edwards TB, Walch G, Sirveaux F, et al. Repair of tears of the subscapularis. J Bone Joint Surg Am 2005;87(4):725–30.

[44] Resch H, Povacz P, Ritter E, et al. Transfer of the pectoralis major muscle for the treatment of irreparable rupture of the subscapularis tendon. J Bone Joint Surg Am 2000;82(3):372–82.

[45] Tolat AR, Amis A, Crofton S, et al. Failure of humeral fracture fixation plate in a young patient using the Philos system: case report. J Shoulder Elbow Surg 2006;15(6):e44–7.

[46] Gerber C, Hersche O, Berberat C. The clinical relevance of posttraumatic avascular necrosis of the humeral head. J Shoulder Elbow Surg 1998;7(6):586–90.

ELSEVIER
SAUNDERS

Orthop Clin N Am 39 (2008) 441–450

ORTHOPEDIC
CLINICS
OF NORTH AMERICA

Hemiarthroplasty for Proximal Humeral Fracture: Restoration of the Gothic Arch

Sumant G. Krishnan, MD*, Phillip W. Bennion, MD, John R. Reineck, MD, Wayne Z. Burkhead, MD

Shoulder and Elbow Service, The Carrell Clinic, 9301 North Central Expressway, Suite 400, Dallas, TX 75231, USA

Historical perspective

Proximal humerus fractures represent 4% to 5% of all fractures and are the most common fractures of the shoulder girdle. Retrospective epidemiologic reviews have demonstrated that proximal humerus fractures accounted for 53% of all significant shoulder girdle injuries [1]. Most of these fractures are the result of a fall, and there is a 2:1 female to male distribution. Furthermore, increasing age has been shown to correlate with increasing fracture risk in women, suggesting an association with osteoporosis. Fractures of the humerus also are the third most common fracture in the elderly (with only hip fractures and Colles' fractures being more common). The incidence of proximal humeral fractures in the elderly has been increasing in recent decades, although the underlying cause for this trend is not clear [2].

Clinical evaluation and indications for treatment

The shoulder girdle often is extremely swollen after a proximal humeral fracture, with ecchymosis often tracking down the arm and into the chest. Because most patients who have proximal humeral fractures are elderly, assessment for concomitant injuries is paramount. Head injuries from the fall, cardiac or neurologic reasons for the fall, and other fractures often are first diagnosed at the initial evaluation for the shoulder injury.

Electromyographic evaluation has demonstrated that approximately two thirds (67%) of all patients who have proximal humeral fractures suffer acute neurologic injury from the violence of the injury. Most commonly, this injury involves either the axillary nerve (58%) and/or the suprascapular nerve (48%). Appreciation and documentation of this finding is important for prognostic evaluation as well as for appropriate management of the injury [3].

Radiographic evaluation

Initial radiographic evaluation consists of the classic Neer trauma series with orthogonal views (anteroposterior, scapular "Y," and axillary views). Because of the anatomy of the proximal humerus, it may be difficult to appreciate fracture lines and fragment displacement. If plain radiographs do not offer adequate visualization, a CT scan with reconstructions may be necessary.

Classification

Neer's four-part classification system of proximal humerus fractures has endured by virtue of its simplicity. It provides a conceptual understanding of the fracture pattern by defining the fracture into separate parts. Interobserver reliability and intraobserver reproducibility have been reported to be only poor to fair, however. Recently, a "comprehensive binary" description of fractures based on Codman's original concept of fracture planes rather than fracture parts has been described [4]. These fracture planes run along the old physeal lines of the proximal humerus. The system results in 12 possible

* Corresponding author.

E-mail address: skrishnan@wbcarrellclinic.com (S.G. Krishnan).

fracture patterns: six patterns resulting in two fracture fragments, five patterns resulting in three fracture fragments, and one pattern resulting in four fracture fragments. This system has demonstrated improved interobserver reliability and better intraobserver reproducibility.

Decision-making algorithm

The peer-reviewed literature is replete with various surgical options for the treatment of proximal humerus fractures. These options include percutaneous fixation with pins and/or screws, arthroscopic-assisted techniques, osteosynthesis with suture and/or plate fixation, intramedullary nail fixation, and arthroplasty. A recent meta-analysis of the surgical management of proximal humerus fractures failed to identify any particular injury in which surgical management would be preferable [5]. Unfortunately, this finding probably resulted from the limited numbers in each patient cohort and the wide variety of injury patterns. There are, however, certain factors that can affect surgical outcomes and therefore influence the choice of surgical technique: age, bone quality, fracture pattern, and timing of surgery (Box 1).

The evidence-based treatment algorithm

Age. Age is the most important consideration in the surgical management of proximal humeral fractures. Fractures in patients aged 70 years or less seem to be more amenable to head/articular surface preservation techniques than fractures in more elderly patients. In patients more than 70 years of age, osteoporotic bone leading to poor fixation as well as poor neuromuscular control may complicate osteosynthesis and lead to unpredictable results because of fixation failure, postoperative fracture displacement/non-union, and/or avascular necrosis.

Bone quality. Bone quality, like age, affects the potential success of any fixation technique that seeks to preserve the native humeral head.

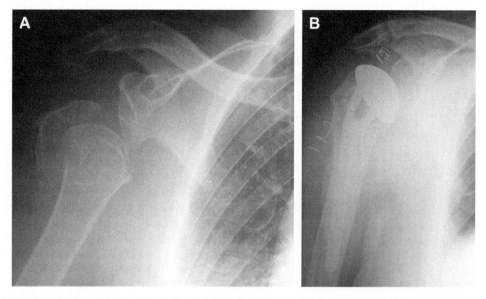

Fig. 1. (*A*) Preoperative anteroposterior radiograph of a proximal humerus fracture. (*B*) Postoperative anteroposterior radiograph of a proximal humerus fracture treated with proximal humeral hemiarthroplasty. (*From* Krishnan SG, Pennington SD, Burkhead WZ, et al. Shoulder arthroplasty for fracture: restoration of the "gothic arch." Techniques in Shoulder and Elbow Surgery 2005;6(2):57–66; with permission.)

Although the development of locking plate technology with angle-stable screws has enhanced the ability to fix fractures in osteoporotic bone, complications remain higher in patients who have weak bone after open reduction internal fixation. Evaluation of the bone mineral density of the proximal humerus and humeral head document higher pullout strengths of cancellous screws in the central region of the humeral head where bone density is highest.

Fracture pattern. When considering head preservation versus replacement for proximal humeral fractures, the question of humeral head viability is paramount. Unfortunately, most of the peer-reviewed literature regarding avascular necrosis after proximal humeral fracture has been studied in a retrospective fashion. Only recently has perfusion of the humeral head after proximal humerus intracapsular fracture been evaluated prospectively [4]. Backflow perfusion of the humeral head was evaluated intraoperatively in this study and then was correlated with preoperative radiographs. It was found that ischemia of the humeral head correlated with certain preoperative radiographic findings. These findings included posteromedial metaphyseal fracture extension of less than 8 mm below the articular surface and disruption of the medial hinge (defined as displacement of the humeral shaft by more than 2 mm). When these two preoperative radiographic findings were present in conjunction with an anatomic neck fracture, there was a 97% positive predictive value for humeral head ischemia. Even when the humeral head is vascular and amenable to preservation, fracture stability still is necessary for successful fracture healing. A requisite intact medial calcar of the humerus therefore is necessary for a stable reduction. Comminution in this region may make fracture stability impossible despite an apparent anatomic reduction.

Timing of surgery. The final variable affecting functional outcome after surgical management of proximal humeral fractures is the delay between injury and definitive surgery. For example, a fracture that initially may be amenable to treatment with percutaneous techniques may become impossible to reduce percutaneously if surgery is delayed too long and early callus prevents achieving that reduction. Similarly, results of arthroplasty for the chronic proximal humeral fractures (> 4 weeks after injury) clearly are different from results of arthroplasty for acute fractures.

Hemiarthroplasty for fracture: restoration of the Gothic arch

Primary hemiarthroplasty for fractures of the proximal humerus can result in good patient satisfaction and pain relief when osteosynthesis is not possible (Fig. 1). A recent retrospective review of 66 patients who underwent hemiarthroplasty for proximal humerus fracture demonstrated that 93% were pain free and satisfied with the results [5]. Similarly, others also have demonstrated successful pain relief but poorer functional outcomes when compared with replacement arthroplasty performed for osteoarthritis.

Recent work has highlighted the importance of intraoperatively restoring anatomic humeral height, humeral version, and tuberosity reconstruction to improve outcomes after arthroplasty for shoulder fracture. The importance of anatomic repositioning of the tuberosities when

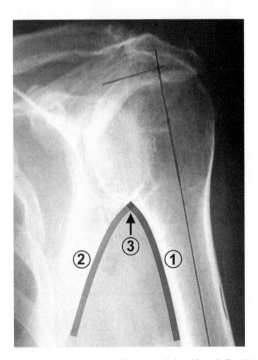

Fig. 2. The Gothic arch of a normal shoulder girdle: (1) Outline the medial border of the proximal humeral shaft ("medial calcar") to the base of the humeral articular surface. (2) Outline the lateral border of the scapula to the base of the glenoid articular surface. (3) Joining these lines creates a classical "vaulted" arch or Gothic arch shape. (*From* Krishnan SG, Pennington SD, Burkhead WZ, et al. Shoulder arthroplasty for fracture: restoration of the "gothic arch." Techniques in Shoulder and Elbow Surgery 2005;6(2):57–66; with permission.)

performing hemiarthroplasty for proximal humeral fracture was demonstrated in a recent cadaveric study [6]. In these cadaveric shoulder specimens, four-part proximal humerus fractures were created and repaired with a shoulder hemiarthroplasty in which the tuberosities were positioned intentionally either anatomically or non-anatomically. The biomechanical effects of this tuberosity positioning demonstrated that anatomic repositioning of the tuberosities around a shoulder hemiarthroplasty produced external rotation kinematics identical to the native shoulder. When the tuberosities were malpositioned, however, an eightfold increase in torque was required to achieve the same degree of external rotation.

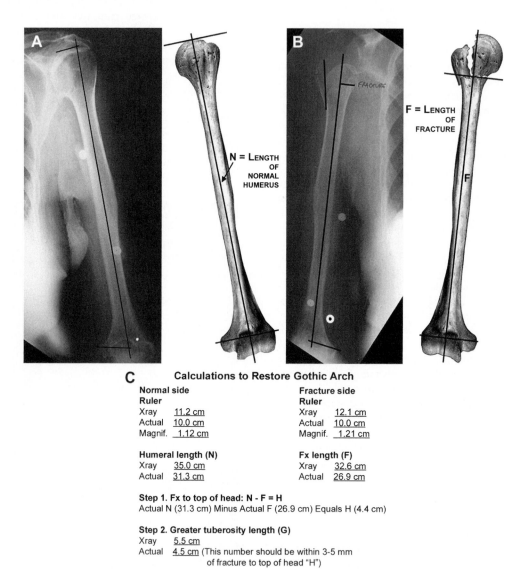

C   Calculations to Restore Gothic Arch

Normal side		Fracture side	
Ruler		**Ruler**	
Xray	11.2 cm	Xray	12.1 cm
Actual	10.0 cm	Actual	10.0 cm
Magnif.	1.12 cm	Magnif.	1.21 cm
Humeral length (N)		**Fx length (F)**	
Xray	35.0 cm	Xray	32.6 cm
Actual	31.3 cm	Actual	26.9 cm

Step 1. Fx to top of head: N - F = H
Actual N (31.3 cm) Minus Actual F (26.9 cm) Equals H (4.4 cm)

Step 2. Greater tuberosity length (G)
Xray   5.5 cm
Actual   4.5 cm (This number should be within 3-5 mm
of fracture to top of head "H")

Fig. 3. (*A*) The length of the normal humerus. N = entire length of normal humerus along perpendicular from medial epicondyle to top of humeral head. A scaled ruler on the radiograph is used to calculate radiographic magnification and obtain the actual number. (*B*) The length of the injured humurus. F = length of injured humerus along perpendicular from medial epicondyle to fracture at superior edge of medial calcar. A scaled ruler on the radiograph is used to calculate radiographic magnification and obtain the actual number. (*C*) Calculations to restore Gothic arch: N − F = H. H is the fracture to top of head height. (*From* Krishnan SG, Pennington SD, Burkhead WZ, et al. Shoulder arthroplasty for fracture: restoration of the "gothic arch." Techniques in Shoulder and Elbow Surgery 2005;6(2):57–66; with permission.)

Clinical studies also have shown that failure to recreate proximal humeral anatomy when treating proximal humerus fractures with hemiarthroplasty can have negative clinical consequences [7]. In these studies, radiographic evidence of final tuberosity malpositioning correlated with poor functional results. Malpositioning of the prosthesis itself in turn correlated with tuberosity malposition. Boileau [8] has pointed out the "unhappy triad" in which a prosthesis not only has excessive height but also is in excessive retroversion and the greater tuberosity has been positioned too low. This combination was associated with poor functional results and persistent pain and stiffness in all cases. It is clear from these studies that careful attention to the recreation of proximal humeral anatomy is critical in shoulder fracture arthroplasty.

The Gothic arch reconstruction

The "Gothic arch" is the term the authors use for the architectural anatomy of the proximal shoulder girdle. The arch is seen easily on a normal radiograph by tracing the medial border of the proximal humeral calcar to the articular surface and joining this line with the lateral border of the scapula to the articular surface: joining these lines forms the classic vaulted or Gothic arch shape seen in Medieval architecture (Fig. 2). Restoration of this Gothic arch provides a very reproducible technique for recreating proper humeral height and improving the potential for reconstruction of the anatomic tuberosity.

Preoperative radiographs are paramount in shoulder fracture arthroplasty and are used to determine the distance from the fracture line at the medial calcar to the desired height of the humeral head. By measuring both the injury films and the contralateral humerus, an accurate assessment of humeral height can be made (Fig. 3A–C). The authors obtain full-length scaled radiographs of the injured and the contralateral humeri with a ruler of defined length. These radiographs even can be obtained in the operating room immediately before surgery and should not be overlooked (Fig. 4A and B). Although in the past surgeons have "eyeballed" the appropriate

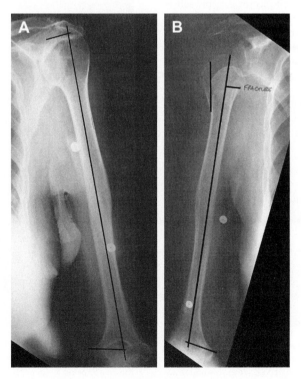

Fig. 4. (*A*) Scaled radiograph of normal humerus. (*B*) Scaled radiograph of injured humerus. (*From* Krishnan SG, Pennington SD, Burkhead WZ, et al. Shoulder arthroplasty for fracture: restoration of the "gothic arch." Techniques in Shoulder and Elbow Surgery 2005;6(2):57–66; with permission.)

prosthetic position subjectively, this simple radiographic preparation allows easy, reproducible, and accurate restoration of proximal humeral anatomy.

In addition, the authors also measure the length of the greater tuberosity fragment to ensure that humeral prosthetic height will allow anatomic tuberosity reconstruction. This measurement is compared with the intraoperative length of the greater tuberosity fragment, which perhaps is the most important measurement, because the greater tuberosity should sit 3 to 5 mm below the prosthetic head.

Surgical technique for restoration of the Gothic arch

The patient is placed in a modified beach-chair position, with the scapula supported. A 2.5- to 3-inch deltopectoral approach is used. The authors have found that a well-placed incision and a mobile soft tissue window permit the procedure to be performed easily through this limited incision (Fig. 5). They begin the incision just below the tip of the coracoid process and parallel the path of the cephalic vein within the deltopectoral interval. This modified deltopectoral approach is medial to traditional shoulder arthroplasty incisions, more horizontal than others describe, and is the incision the authors use for all fracture and primary shoulder arthroplasties. With

adequate exposure, the fracture is visualized. Typically the fracture line can be located with a blunt elevator or osteotome between the tuberosities, just posterior to the bicipital groove. Four horizontal mattress nonabsorbable sutures are placed around the greater tuberosity at the bone–tendon junction (two in the infraspinatus and two in the teres minor). Two temporary stay sutures are placed around the lesser tuberosity at the subscapularis/bone tendon junction. The tuberosities are retracted apart gently. The head fragment is removed and measured with a caliper. If the fractured humeral head measures between prosthetic sizes, the smaller of the two prosthetic head sizes is selected. Structural cancellous bone graft is procured from this articular fragment.

The medullary canal is prepared using cylindrical reamers by hand and fracture-specific trial implants (Aequalis Fracture Prosthesis, Tornier, St. Ismier, France) of increasing diameter. Once the appropriate trial implant and head size are determined, retroversion is selected by facing the

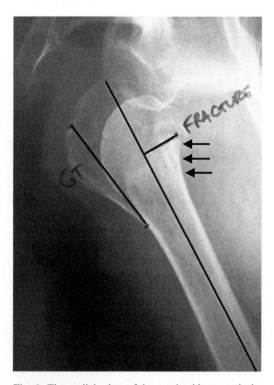

Fig. 6. The medial calcar of the proximal humerus is the portion of the humeral shaft just below the inferior limit of the anatomic neck. (*From* Krishnan SG, Pennington SD, Burkhead WZ, et al. Shoulder arthroplasty for fracture: restoration of the "gothic arch." Techniques in Shoulder and Elbow Surgery 2005;6(2):57–66; with permission.)

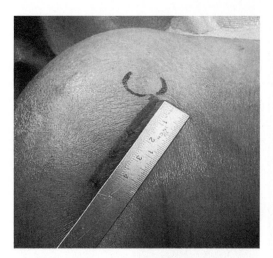

Fig. 5. Limited 3-inch modified deltopectoral incision used for shoulder fracture arthroplasty. (*From* Krishnan SG, Pennington SD, Burkhead WZ, et al. Shoulder arthroplasty for fracture: restoration of the "gothic arch." Techniques in Shoulder and Elbow Surgery 2005;6(2):57–66; with permission.)

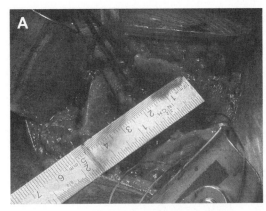

B Calculations to Restore Gothic Arch

Normal side		Fracture side	
Ruler		**Ruler**	
Xray	11.2 cm	Xray	12.1 cm
Actual	10.0 cm	Actual	10.0 cm
Magnif.	1.12 cm	Magnif.	1.21 cm

Humeral length (N)		Fx length (F)	
Xray	35.0 cm	Xray	32.6 cm
Actual	31.3 cm	Actual	26.9 cm

Step 1. Fx to top of head: N - F = H
Actual N (31.3 cm) Minus Actual F (26.9 cm) Equals H (4.4 cm)

Step 2. Greater tuberosity length (G)
Xray 5.5 cm
Actual 4.5 cm (This number should be within 3-5 mm
of fracture to top of head "H")

Step 3. Greater tuberosity measurement
Measurement 4.6 cm (This number should be within 5 mm
of greater tuberosity length "G")

Fig. 7. (*A*) Greater tuberosity length (G in Fig. 7B) is measured and corrected for radiographic magnification using a scale on the radiograph. (*B*) The length of the greater tuberosity (G) should be within 3 to 5 mm of the fracture to top of head height (H) that was marked on the prosthetic implant. (*From* Krishnan SG, Pennington SD, Burkhead WZ, et al. Shoulder arthroplasty for fracture: restoration of the "gothic arch." Techniques in Shoulder and Elbow Surgery 2005;6(2):57–66; with permission.)

prosthetic head toward the glenoid with the forearm in neutral rotation at the side (approximately 20° of retroversion relative to the transepicondylar axis of the elbow).

The dedicated fracture-specific prosthetic stem of the appropriate diameter is opened, and the preselected trial head is placed on this definitive implant with the eccentric head offset rotated into the most lateral position. This placement allows for the least amount of medial overhang of the prosthetic head during the all-important restoration of the Gothic arch.

This surgical technique differs from previously described techniques that reference the prosthetic humeral reconstruction off of the lateral portion of the humerus and humeral metadiaphysis. In most proximal humeral fractures, the medial calcar of the proximal humerus (the proximal medial humeral shaft just inferior to the anatomic neck) is intact (Fig. 6). In the few cases in which

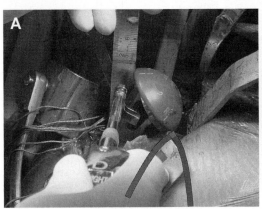

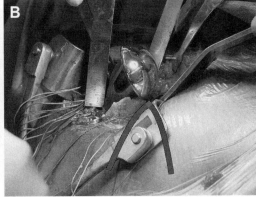

Fig. 8. (*A*) Gothic arch restoration with trial head on actual implant. Implant has been placed to predetermined mark and confirmed with ruler. (*B*) Final Gothic arch restoration. (*From* Krishnan SG, Pennington SD, Burkhead WZ, et al. Shoulder arthroplasty for fracture: restoration of the "gothic arch." Techniques in Shoulder and Elbow Surgery 2005;6(2):57–66; with permission.)

the medial calcar is fractured, this fragment often is large and can be fixed rigidly with simple wire or heavy suture fixation. By referencing the reconstruction off of the medial calcar, the Gothic arch can be recreated objectively in a methodical fashion (Fig. 7A and B).

Using the preoperative radiographic calculations as described previously, the appropriate mark is placed on the prosthetic implant, and the implant is placed into the humeral shaft with the appropriately selected trial head. The lateral half of the Gothic arch (medial calcar of the humerus up to the inferior margin of the anatomic neck) should be unbroken (Fig. 8A and B). If the arch is not visualized, then (1) the prosthetic height is incorrect (usually too high), (2) the medial calcar is fractured and has not been restored, or (3) the head is too large or has not been rotated into the most lateral offset position.

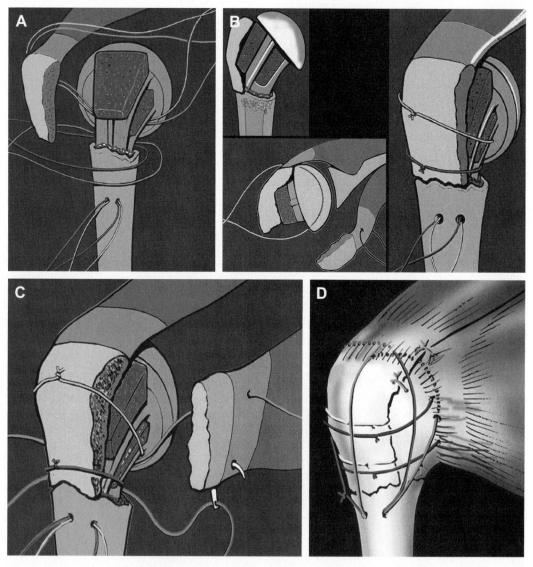

Fig. 9. (*A*) Six-suture configuration for anatomic tuberosity osteosynthesis. (*B*) Greater tuberosity fixation over lateral bone graft. (*C*) Lesser tuberosity fixation over medial bone graft. (*D*) Final tuberosity osteosynthesis with tension-band sutures passed through anterosuperior and posterosuperior cuff. (*From* Krishnan SG, Pennington SD, Burkhead WZ, et al. Shoulder arthroplasty for fracture: restoration of the "gothic arch." Techniques in Shoulder and Elbow Surgery 2005;6(2):57–66; with permission.)

After the arch is established, two drill holes are placed in the proximal humeral shaft before final prosthetic cementation. Two nonabsorbable sutures are placed in these holes in a horizontal mattress fashion to be used as tension-band sutures for final tuberosity osteosynthesis. The stem is cemented using a standard third-generation technique to the predetermined depth and rotation, in slight valgus. Three structural cancellous bone graft wedges that were obtained previously from the fractured humeral head are placed (1) in the window of the fracture-specific prosthesis, (2) under the greater tuberosity at the lateral fin of the prosthesis, and (3) under the medial edge of the prosthetic head between the head and neck of the implant.

Tuberosity osteosynthesis is performed as described elsewhere, and the biceps is tenodesed within the intertubercular groove/rotator interval to soft tissue (Fig. 9A–D) [8,9]. The shoulder is placed through a full range of motion to ensure there is no micromotion of the tuberosity fragments. Passive intraoperative range of motion should be at least 160° of elevation, 40° of external rotation, and 70° of internal rotation. Postoperative radiographs should demonstrate anatomic reconstruction of the proximal humerus (see Fig. 1).

Postoperatively, patients are placed into a SmartSling orthosis (Innovation Sports/Ossur, Aliso Viejo, California) for 6 weeks. Immediate supine passive motion is begun the day after surgery with motion limits dictated by the intraoperative evaluation following tuberosity osteosynthesis. Active motion is allowed 7 weeks after surgery. Resistance exercises begin 10 weeks after surgery.

Clinical results after shoulder hemiarthroplasty for fracture

The authors have reviewed retrospectively 130 consecutive patients who had proximal humerus fractures and who underwent the Gothic arch restoration technique for fracture arthroplasty at a minimum 2-year follow-up [9]. Mean active anterior elevation (AAE) was 129° (range, 50°–165°), the mean American Shoulder and Elbow Surgeons' (ASES) score was 74 (range, 10–100), and 114 (88%) greater tuberosities healed anatomically. Pain scores averaged 1.2 on a scale on which zero represented no pain and 10 represented the worst pain possible. Satisfaction averaged 9.1 on a scale on which zero indicated unsatisfied and 10 represented completely satisfied. For patients who had AAE greater than 120° (106 cases), the mean age was 62 years, the mean AAE was 146°, the mean ASES score was 86, and 94% of tuberosities healed. Patients who had an AAE of less than 120° (24 cases) had a mean age of 82 years, a mean AAE of 95°, a mean ASES score of 46, and 61% of the tuberosities healed ($P < .03$). For patients who had fracture-specific prosthesis (65 cases), the mean AAE was 140°, the mean ASES score was 82, and 92% of tuberosities healed ($P < .05$) [9].

Summary

Four-part proximal humerus fractures represent a difficult entity in the management of upper extremity trauma. Most of these fractures are not amenable to head-preserving osteosynthesis techniques, so surgical management usually involves head-replacing fracture arthroplasty. Timely reestablishment of the Gothic arch using a fracture-specific prosthesis reliably leads to anatomic tuberosity osteosynthesis. Hence, shoulder arthroplasty for fracture should be considered an augmented osteosynthesis, with precise prosthetic implantation supplementing anatomic tuberosity reconstruction. Investigations regarding the use of specific fracture implants and biologic substrates are ongoing in an attempt to improve further the rate of tuberosity healing after this operation in older patients.

References

[1] Nordqvist A, Petersson CJ. Incidence and causes of shoulder girdle injuries in an urban population. J Shoulder Elbow Surg 1995;4(2):107–12.

[2] Palvanen M, Kannus P, Niemi S, et al. Update in the epidemiology of proximal humeral fractures. Clin Orthop Relat Res 2006;442:87–92.

[3] Visser CP, Coene LN, Brand R, et al. Nerve lesions in proximal humeral fractures. J Shoulder Elbow Surg 2001;10(5):421–7.

[4] Hertel R, Hempfing A, Stiehler M, et al. Predictors of humeral head ischemia after intracapsular fracture of the proximal humerus. J Shoulder Elbow Surg 2004;13(4):427–33.

[5] Mighell MA, Kolm GP, Collinge CA, et al. Outcomes of hemiarthroplasty for fractures of the proximal humerus. J Shoulder Elbow Surg 2003;12(6):569–77.

[6] Frankle MA, Greenwald DP, Markee BA, et al. Biomechanical effects of malposition of tuberosity fragments on the humeral prosthetic reconstruction for four-part proximal humerus fractures. J Shoulder Elbow Surg 2001;10(4):321–6.

[7] Boileau P, Krishnan SG, Tinsi L, et al. Tuberosity malposition and migration: reasons for poor outcomes after hemiarthroplasty for displaced fractures of the proximal humerus. J Shoulder Elbow Surg 2002;11(5):401–12.

[8] Boileau P, Walch G, Krishnan SG. Tuberosity osteosynthesis and hemiarthroplasty for four-part fractures of the proximal humerus. Techniques in Shoulder and Elbow Surgery 2000;1:96–109.

[9] Krishnan SG, Lin KC, Burkhead WZ. Shoulder arthroplasty for fracture: results of the Gothic arch technique and a fracture-specific prosthesis. Presented at American Shoulder and Elbow Surgeons Specialty Day Proceedings. San Diego, California, March 8, 2007.

ELSEVIER
SAUNDERS

Orthop Clin N Am 39 (2008) 451–457

ORTHOPEDIC
CLINICS
OF NORTH AMERICA

Reverse Total Shoulder Arthroplasty for Acute Fractures and Failed Management After Proximal Humeral Fractures

Thomas G. Martin, BS[a], Joseph P. Iannotti, MD, PhD[b],*

[a]Case Western Reserve University, School of Medicine, 10900 Euclid Avenue, Cleveland, OH 44106, USA
[b]Department of Orthopaedic Surgery, Cleveland Clinic, A-41, 9500 Euclid Avenue, Cleveland, OH 44195, USA

Proximal humeral fractures (PHFs), representing the second most common fracture of the upper extremity [1], continue to increase in number as the number of elderly in the population increases [2]. One epidemiologic survey of the United States Medicare population found that PHFs account for 10% of all fractures in patients 65 years or older [3]. Most PHFs are minimally displaced or nondisplaced and have noncontroversial treatment modalities. Surgical treatment options for at least 15% of the remaining PHFs range from closed reduction and percutaneous pinning to open reduction and internal fixation or prosthetic replacement.

Complex three- and four-part fractures are shown to be difficult to manage with surgical reconstruction, particularly when combined with significant comminution of the fragments, dislocation of the articular segment, and osteoporosis. Avascular necrosis of the articular head fragment is common and experience has shown that prosthetic replacement is appropriate in many cases of four-part fractures in the elderly with the exception of the valgus-impacted type, which may better preserve blood supply to the humeral head [4].

Hemiarthroplasty as a primary treatment of complex PHF has achieved mixed results. Early work by Neer [5] and associates showed excellent pain relief and restoration of function. More recent studies, however, have demonstrated acceptable pain relief but varying functional outcomes [6]. Results often are complicated by failure of tuberosity osteosynthesis, resulting in malunion or nonunions, poor initial position of the prosthesis, or inadequate reduction of the greater tuberosity, with each of these complications made more frequent in the presence of osteopenia [7]. Loss of fixation of the tuberosities with malunion or nonunion can cause a deficient or nonfunctional rotator cuff with or without glenohumeral arthritis.

The reverse shoulder arthroplasty (RSA) converts the humeral head into a socket and the glenoid into a convex articulating surface. In this design, the articular surfaces are constrained resulting in a fixed center of rotation. In addition, the moment arm and length of the deltoid muscle are increased. The reverse shoulder design increases the deltoid moment arm by medializing the center of rotation and by shifting the deltoid insertion site distally. These two factors make the centering function of the rotator cuff less important for shoulder elevation and improve the mechanical advantage of the deltoid. Both factors result in an improvement in shoulder function in the presence of an insufficient rotator cuff.

The reverse total shoulder prosthesis designed by Paul Grammont originally was intended to manage glenohumeral arthritis in the setting of rotator cuff insufficiency. Intermediate-term experience has shown promising results in elderly patients who have cuff tear arthropathy [8]. Clinical experience has extended the use of this

---

* Corresponding author. Cleveland Clinic, Department of Orthopaedic Surgery A-41, 9500 Euclid Avenue, Cleveland OH 44195.

E-mail address: iannotj@ccf.org (J.P. Iannotti).

prosthetic device for management of acute complex PHFs in the very elderly and treatment of sequelae of PHFs where distortion of the proximal humeral anatomy (malunion and nonunion of the tuberosities) results in a dysfunctional rotator cuff.

Reverse shoulder arthroplasty for acute proximal humeral fractures

A few small series exist regarding treatment of acute PHF with RSA, and the level of evidence to date regarding such treatment remains low. Bufquin and colleagues observed 43 patients, mean age 78 years, who had been treated with RSA for three- or four-part PHF with a mean follow-up of 22 months. Clinical outcomes included an active anterior elevation of 97° and an active external rotation in abduction of 30°. The postoperative Constant Shoulder Score was 44 and the mean modified Constant score was 66% [9].

Another small series of 15 patients (mean age 78 years) was reported from a large 457 case multicenter study of reverse arthroplasty. Three cases were described as three-part displaced fractures with humeral head and lesser tuberosity displacement, and 12 cases were classified as four-part displaced fractures. Average follow-up was 46 months; the mean active anterior elevation was 107° and external rotation was 10°. The investigators observed recovery of active external rotation when the tuberosity healed, but the trend was not statistically significant given the small number of cases. Also, the mean Constant score was 55 points. The investigators compared their data with data from hemiarthroplasty treatment cases. Mean active elevation in the reverse group was similar to that observed in the hemiarthroplasty group. The distributions in active anterior elevation varied, however, between reverse and hemiarthroplasty groups. In the reverse group, only one patient had less than 90° active anterior elevation but the anterior elevation never exceeded 150°. The anterior elevation in the hemiarthroplasty group, however, was more skewed with 50% of patients attaining 90° or less and 11% having more than 150° active anterior elevation. In terms of Constant score, the hemiarthroplasty group outcome was heavily dependent on tuberosity healing. When the greater tuberosity did not heal, the mean Constant score was 55 points for the reverse prosthesis group and 41 for hemiarthroplasty group.

Similarly, active anterior elevation was 75° in the hemiarthroplasty group and 116° in the reverse group in cases of malunion or nonunion of the greater tuberosity [10].

Cazeneuve and Cristofari reported on a series of 23 patients treated with reverse arthroplasty for acute PHF. The mean follow-up was 86 months and the mean age 75 years. Excluding two cases that required revision, the postoperative active anterior elevation was greater than 120°and the mean Constant score was 60 points in the remaining cases. Radiographically, tuberosities were displaced in 53% of cases. Furthermore, the investigators observed a more complete recovery of active external rotation when the tuberosities had been fixed [11].

The authors' experience with use of the reverse total shoulder for acute fractures has been limited to a few cases. Its use for this indication should be limited to older and sedentary patients. The results have been encouraging (Fig. 1).

Reverse shoulder arthroplasty for proximal humeral nonunion and malunion

Relatively few data are available concerning pain and function outcomes after reverse arthroplasty as treatment of fracture sequelae. In a series of 45 patients, mean age 72 years and mean follow-up of 39 months, Neyton and coworkers observed improvement in active elevation from 59° to 114° while noting no significant change in external rotation. Constant scores improved from 20 to 53 with postoperative shoulder function improving to 75% of normal shoulder function for the same age and gender [12].

Neyton and associates reviewed their clinical experience with RSA as a treatment of different types of fracture sequelae. Fracture sequelae were categorized into four types. Patients who had cephalic collapse of the humeral head (type 1) had equivalent results to RSA when compared with the use of a nonconstrained prosthesis. Patients treated with hemiarthroplasty had better external rotation function when compared with patients treated with RSA. This may be related to medialization of the center of rotation, with RSA, resulting in shortening of the external rotators. Therefore, with humeral head collapse and intact tuberosities, it is best to use a nonconstrained prosthesis. When the tuberosities are severely displaced and the rotator cuff is nonfunctional before surgery, then a RSA is best. For locked or fracture dislocations (type 2), either option could be used although RSA was

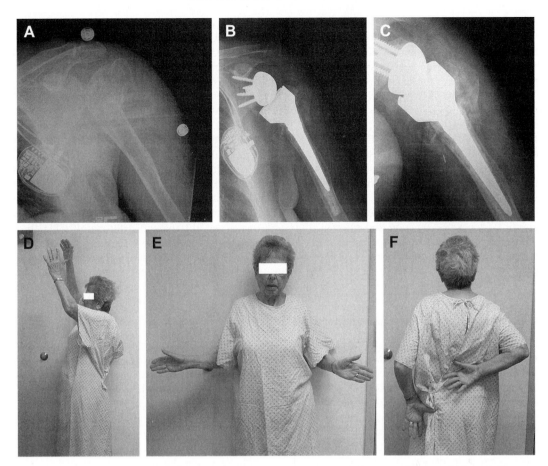

Fig. 1. An 82-year-old woman who had an acute four-part fracture with significant cardiac comorbidity (*A*). Two-year follow-up radiographs (*B*, *C*); tuberosities have healed around the prosthesis and clinical result (*D*, *E*, *F*).

preferred for chronic anterior dislocation because nonconstrained prostheses did not adequately stabilize this type of dislocation. For humeral surgical neck nonunion (type 3), RSA was observed to have a high complication rate similar to that observed for nonconstrained treatment. Nonarthroplasty treatment consisting of intramedullary bone peg graft and internal fixation was recommended by these investigators. Finally, unlike nonconstrained prostheses, RSA treatment of severe distortion of proximal humeral anatomy with malunion (type 4) was shown to give acceptable pain and function results despite postoperative nonunion or malunion of the greater tuberosity.

Reverse shoulder arthroplasty for failed hemiarthroplasty

Several recent studies have reported on the operative experience of management of failed hemiarthroplasty for complex PHF using RSA. Levy and associates reported on a series of 29 patients who had failed hemiarthroplasty who underwent a single-stage revision to a reverse prosthesis with mean follow-up time of 35 months. Improvement was seen in forward flexion by an average of 34.6° and in abduction by 36.3°. Increases in Simple Shoulder Test and American Shoulder and Elbow Surgeons (ASES) scores also were observed. Patients who had proximal humeral bone loss were divided into those treated with a reverse shoulder prosthesis alone and those treated with a proximal humeral allograft–reverse shoulder prosthesis construct. An improvement in functional scores (with the exception of forward elevation) was observed in patients who had been treated with a reverse shoulder prosthesis combined with a proximal humeral allograft [13].

Another study, conducted by Boileau and colleagues, identified 45 patients who received the Grammont Delta III prosthesis (DePuy, Warsaw, Indiana) for varying indications with a mean follow-up of 40 months. Nineteen of the 45 patients, mean age 67 years, received a revision reverse arthroplasty for failed hemiarthroplasty. The improvement in anterior elevation in the revision series (56° to 113°) was similar to the improvement observed in the cuff tear arthropathy series (53° to 123°). The improvement in adjusted ASES scores and Constant scores for revision patients, however, was significantly less than that for similarly treated cuff tear arthropathy patients. An improvement in external or internal rotation was not observed in the revision group. Postoperative function and external rotation were correlated with postoperative external rotation strength and absence of a hornblower's sign [14].

Complications after reverse shoulder arthroplasty

Complications after reverse arthroplasty for various indications are reported in many studies. Bufquin and associates observed that the major difficulty after treatment of acute PHF with RSA was fixation of tuberosities resulting in malunions or nonunions. Tuberosities remained intact in 17 of 40 patients available for radiologic review (42.5%). The effect on the Constant score seemed moderate. A 28% (12 out of 43 cases) complication rate was reported in this study and complications included one perioperative glenoid fracture, five transient neurologic complications, three cases of reflex sympathetic dystrophy, one secondary deltoid rupture, one acromion fracture, and one dislocation. These complication trends, as the investigators point out, also are observed in studies of treating acute fracture with hemiarthroplasty [15,16]. Cazeneuve and Cristofari [11] reported four similar complications, including two cases of reflex sympathetic dystrophy, one dislocation, and one infection. The latter two complications required revision surgery.

Significant complications also are observed in patients treated with reverse arthroplasty for fracture sequelae. Neyton and associates observed a 23% complication rate, the most common complication being postoperative deep infection (9.3%). The high rate of infection is related to the revision nature of this surgery in an elderly patient population. Other complications reported were painful persistent stiffness, periprosthetic fracture,

anterior dislocation, intraoperative glenoid fracture, and axillary nerve palsy [12].

Postoperative complications of reverse arthroplasty performed for failed hemiarthroplasty also have been observed in different studies. Levy and associates observed complications in 8 of the 28 patients followed in their study (28%). In their proximal humeral allograft–reverse shoulder prosthesis group, complications occurred in three of eight patients and included postoperative infection, dislocation, and periprosthetic fracture from a fall [13]. Boileau and colleagues [14] noted a substantially higher complication rate (47%) in the failed hemiarthroplasty group than in patients treated for rotator cuff arthropathy (5%). In a multicenter study of 457 cases of reverse arthroplasty, Walch and associates observed a complication rate of 25% for RSA as a revision for failed hemiarthroplasty. Furthermore, they pointed out that RSA used in revision surgery has a complication rate three times as high as that of primary RSA [17].

Although RSA is able to restore active elevation, little or no improvement in external rotation is a common outcome because this prosthetic cannot substitute for the external rotation function of the posterior part of the rotator cuff. In addition, the center of rotation is medialized, decreasing the effectiveness of the posterior deltoid as a secondary external rotator when coupled with abduction. Lastly, passive external rotation is hampered by the inherent design of the reverse prosthesis resulting in impingement of the components at the limits of their articulating surfaces (Fig. 2) [14].

The frequency of scapular notching is a cause for concern in RSA in general and it is no less the case for treatment of fracture sequelae and acute fracture. Neyton observed notching of the inferior part of the scapular neck in 14 (37%) of 38 available follow-up radiographs, with notching extending beyond the inferior screw in five cases (grades 3 and 4). Although notching was observed in a significant portion of the study participants, it was not attributed to have a negative effect on pain, functional scoring, or complications [12]. Notching after treatment of acute fracture also has been observed. Bufquin and colleagues [9] reported scapular notching in 69% of cases and in one case a metaglene became loose. Although glenoid notching is a concern for long-term stability of the glenoid component of RSA, the phenomenon may be of less significance in this group of elderly patients.

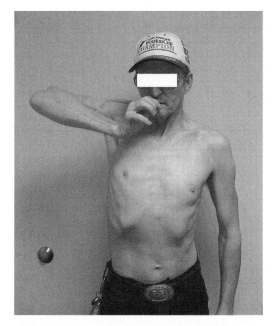

Fig. 2. A 72-year-old man treated with RSA for failed total shoulder arthroplasty with a postoperative positive hornblower's sign. Patient is satisfied with the clinical result but external rotation may have been improved by use of a latissiumus dorsi transfer at the time of revision to a reverse arthroplasty.

Disease/Surgery (Group)	# patients	Average Age (Range)	% Male
OA/TSA	144	68.0 (38 – 89)	55
CTA/Hemi	31	69.9 (50 – 84)	29
CTA/Reverse	43	70.9 (35 – 88)	41
Hemi/Reverse	21	66.1 (45 – 84)	42

Fig. 3. One hundred forty-four patients who had primary osteoarthritis had a total shoulder arthroplasty (OA/TSA) using a Global Advantage (DePuy Johnson and Johnson, Warsaw, Indiana). Thirty-one patients who had primary rotator cuff tear arthropathy had a hemiarthroplasty (CTA/Hemi) performed using a DePuy CTA humeral head (DePuy Johnson and Johnson). Forty-three patients who had rotator cuff tear arthropathy underwent replacement (CTA/Reverse) with a Delta III reverse total shoulder (DePuy Johnson and Johnson). Twenty-one patients had failed hemiarthroplasty for treatment of PHFs and were revised to a Delta reverse total shoulder arthroplasty (Hemi/Reverse). The average age, age range, and percent male patients in each group are shown.

Authors' clinical experience with reverse shoulder arthroplasty for fracture sequelae and failed hemiarthroplasty for proximal humeral fracture

Anatomic total shoulder arthroplasty for treatment of osteoarthritis in patients who have an intact rotator cuff is a gold standard for comparing the quality of the result of treatment of other forms of arthritis by prosthetic arthroplasty. The Cleveland Clinic shoulder arthroplasty database (Fig. 3) demonstrates that the results of anatomic total shoulder arthroplasty for osteoarthritis resulted in sustained improvement in functional outcome and pain relief with a shoulder score of 80 of a possible 100 points. In this cohort, 93% of patients were improved after surgery, with 79% having postoperative scores more than 30 points improved over preoperative levels.

Rotator cuff tear arthropathy presents other challenges as patients generally are older and have more comorbidity and lower short form-12 scores for general medical health. The use of hemiarthroplasty usually results in good pain relief but variable improvement in function (Fig. 4). Eighty-two percent of patients had at least a 15-point

improvement in their postoperative shoulder scores but only 50% had at least a 30-point improvement.

Improvement in pain and functional outcome clearly is better with reverse total shoulder arthroplasty, with scores on average 10 points

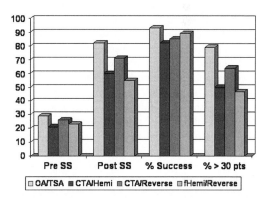

Fig. 4. The patients in each group (see table Fig. 3) were followed using the University of Pennsylvania Shoulder Score (maximum total score 100 points). Results shown are at a minimum of 1 year after surgery. Percent successful outcome (% success) is defined as the percentage of patients that achieve at least a 15-point improvement in their shoulder scores over their preoperative scores. The percentage of patients who had greater than a 30-point improvement in postoperative score are shown for each patient group.

better than hemiarthoplasty for total postoperative scores. Eighty-five percent of patients have at least a 15-point improvement and 64% at least a 30-point improvement. When comparing the subscores between hemiarthroplasty and reverse total shoulder arthroplasty for treatment of primary rotator cuff tear arthropathy, the difference in results primarily are the result of better function in the reverse arthroplasty groups.

Reverse total shoulder arthroplasty is indicated for the management of failed hemiarthroplasty for PHF in the presence of rotator cuff deficiency. The results are improved from preoperative status in 89% of patients, and 47% of patients had at least a 30-point improvement over preoperative scores. Postoperative and preoperative overall shoulder scores were the lowest of any other group of patients demonstrating the severity of the shoulder problems and functional disability that exist in these patients and the salvage nature of this surgery. Nonetheless, reverse total shoulder replacement offers these patients an opportunity for improvement in pain and function that no other reconstructive surgery can offer.

Summary

RSA has a highly successful clinical record when used for treatment of arthropathy accompanied by rotator cuff insufficiency, as demonstrated in several studies [8,18,19]. Based on this experience, efforts to use the same technology for other conditions involving insufficient cuff function have been described but, to date, have had limited results reported in the literature. Two conditions related to PHF described in this review for which RSA has shown promise seem to be treatment of failed hemiarthroplasty and treatment of complex fracture sequelae, such as tuberosity or surgical neck nonunion and malunion, avascular necrosis, and locked dislocation. Because experience is limited, specific conclusions as yet are difficult to reach. Thus far, it seems clear that the amount of remaining cuff tissue and surgical technique, especially accuracy of component placement, are critically important in treatment of cases of failed hemiarthroplasty and fracture sequelae, which parallels the experience of RSA in the treatment of rotator cuff tear arthropathy. The cumulative experience to date also suggests that results show improvement in pain levels, and the incidence of complications only mimics that of cases of major revision shoulder surgery

in general, namely, fewer satisfactory results with greater complication rates than are seen in primary procedures. Pain relief, however, is more reliably gained than is return of strength or shoulder function and the types of complications are not necessarily unique or trendworthy. That is, given the unique arthroplasty procedure performed and when using appropriate surgical technique, no inherent complication seems to prevail, such as loosening, instability, or infection. Success with RSA, when used for treatment of failed hemiarthroplasty or fracture sequelae, as in the case of revision surgery in general, seems related to the quality of the remaining tissues. This includes sufficient and compliant subscapularis, deltoid, and teres minor muscles, along with adequate glenohumeral bone stock. When coupled with sound surgical technique for proper placement of the components and good fixation to bone, RSA provides for deltoid-driven elevation and pain relief in most patients. Some patients may still experience limited active external rotation. Future studies are needed to determine if supplemental soft tissue procedures (eg, latissimus dorsi transfer) or modification of the implant design will serve to improve functional outcome in this difficult-to-treat subset of patients.

References

[1] Baron JA, Barrett JA, Karagas MR. The epidemiology of peripheral fractures. Bone 1996;18(3 Suppl): 209S–13S.

[2] Hodgson S. Proximal humerus fracture rehabilitation. Clin Orthop Relat Res 2006;442:131–8.

[3] Baron JA, Karagas M, Barrett J, et al. Basic epidemiology of fractures of the upper and lower limb among Americans over 65 years of age. Epidemiology 1996;7:612–8.

[4] Naranja RJ Jr, Iannotti JP. Displaced three- and four-part proximal humerus fractures: evaluation and management. J Am Acad Orthop Surg 2000; 8(6):373–82.

[5] Neer CS II. Displaced proximal humeral fractures. I. classification and evaluation. J Bone Joint Surg Am 1970;52(6):1077–89.

[6] Tanner MW, Cofield RH. Prosthetic arthroplasty for fractures and fracture-dislocations of the proximal humerus. Clin Orthop Relat Res 1983;179: 116–28.

[7] Boileau P, Krishnan SG, Tinsi L, et al. Tuberosity malposition and migration: reasons for poor outcomes after hemiarthroplasty for displaced fractures of the proximal humerus. J Shoulder Elbow Surg 2002;11(5):401–12.

[8] Favard L, Le Du C, Bicknell R, et al. Reverse prosthesis for cuff tear arthritis (Hamada IV and V) without previous surgery. In: Walch G, Boileau P, Mole D, editors. Reverse shoulder arthroplasty, clinical results—complications—revision. Montpellier (France): Sauramps Medical; 2006. p. 113–23.

[9] Bufquin T, Hersan A, Hubert L, et al. Reverse shoulder arthroplasty for the treatment of three- and four-part fractures of the proximal humerus in the elderly: a prospective review of 43 cases with a short-term follow-up. J Bone Joint Surg Br 2007;89(4):516–20.

[10] Sirveaux F, Navez GN, Favard L, et al. Reverse prosthesis for acute proximal humerus fracture, the multicentric study. In: Walch G, Boileau P, Mole D, et al, editors. Reverse shoulder arthroplasty, clinical results—complications—revision. Montpellier (France): Sauramps Médical; 2006. p. 73–80.

[11] Cazeneuve JF, Cristofari DJ. Grammont reversed prosthesis for acute complex fracture of the proximal humerus in an elderly population with 5 to 12 years follow-up. Rev Chir Orthop Reparatrice Appar Mot 2006;92(6):543–8.

[12] Neyton L, Garaud P, Boileau P, et al. Results of reverse shoulder arthroplasty in proximal humerus fracture sequelae. In: Walch G, Boileau P, Mole D, et al, editors. Reverse shoulder arthroplasty, clinical results—complications—revision. Montpellier (France): Sauramps Médical; 2006. p. 81–101.

[13] Levy J, Frankle M, Mighell M, et al. The use of the reverse shoulder prosthesis for the treatment of failed hemiarthroplasty for proximal humeral fracture. J Bone Joint Surg Am 2007;89(2):292–300.

[14] Boileau P, Watkinson D, Hatzidakis AM, et al. Neer Award 2005: the Grammont reverse shoulder prosthesis: results in cuff tear arthritis, fracture sequelae, and revision arthroplasty. J Shoulder Elbow Surg 2006;15(5):527–40.

[15] Boileau P, Trojani C, Walch G, et al. Shoulder arthroplasty for the treatment of the sequelae of fractures of the proximal humerus. J Shoulder Elbow Surg 2001;10(4):299–308.

[16] Neer CS 2nd, McIlveen SJ. Humeral head replacement with reconstruction of the tuberosities and the cuff in 4-fragment displaced fractures. Current results and technics. Rev Chir Orthop Reparatrice Appar Mot 1988;74(Suppl 2):31–40.

[17] Walch G, Wall B, Mottier F. Complications and revision of the reverse prosthesis: a multicenter study of 457 cases. In: Walch G, Boileau P, Mole D, editors. Reverse shoulder arthroplasty, clinical results—complications—revision. Montpellier (France): Sauramps Medical; 2006. p. 335–52.

[18] Baulot E, Chabernaud D, Grammont P. Results of Grammont's inverted prosthesis in omarthritis associated with major cuff destruction: apropos of 16 cases. Acta Orthop Belg 1995;61:112–9.

[19] Sirveaux F, Favard L, Oudet D, et al. Grammont inverted total shoulder arthroplasty in the treatment of glenohumeral osteoarthritis with massive rupture of the cuff. Results of a multicenter study of 80 shoulders. J Bone Joint Surg Br 2004;86:388–95.

ORTHOPEDIC
CLINICS
OF NORTH AMERICA

Orthop Clin N Am 39 (2008) 459–474

Scapula Fractures

Peter C. Lapner, MD, FRCSC[a],*, Hans K. Uhthoff, MD, FRCSC[a],
Steve Papp, MD, FRCSC[b]

[a]Division of Orthopedics, University of Ottawa, The Ottawa Hospital, 1648 Critical Care Wing,
Box 502, 501 Smyth Road, Ottawa, Ontario, Canada K1H 8L6
[b]Division of Orthopedics, University of Ottawa, The Ottawa Hospital, 1053 Carling Avenue,
Ottawa, Ontario, Canada K1Y 4E9

Fractures of the scapula are relatively rare injuries; they represent 3% to 5% of all fractures involving the shoulder girdle and 1% of fractures overall [1,2]. The rarity of the injury is likely because of the thick soft tissue envelope that surrounds the scapula. In addition, some protection is conferred by the mobility of the glenohumeral articulation and other joints that make up the shoulder complex, including the acromioclavicular joint, the sternoclavicular joint, and the scapulothoracic interface.

Glenoid and scapular body fractures typically occur secondary to high-energy trauma and thus are most commonly seen in young and middle-aged males. Direct trauma to the lateral or posterosuperior aspect of the forequarter is the most common mechanism of injury. Ninety percent of patients who sustain scapular fractures have other associated injuries [3,4]. Because attention is often directed initially toward these other injuries, fractures of the scapula are often initially overlooked.

Because fractures of the scapula are rare and the diagnosis and treatment may be unfamiliar to some surgeons, this article outlines a diagnostic work-up and treatment approach for the various types of scapular fractures. The approach helps guide decision making on operative versus nonoperative treatment based on what is known regarding prognosis and outcomes of management. Operative technique and fixation strategies are discussed for the common fracture patterns along with guidelines for postsurgical shoulder rehabilitation.

Anatomy

A thorough knowledge of scapular anatomy is required to appreciate the nature and complexity of scapular fractures. An understanding of the various muscle attachments and bony contours is a prerequisite for planning surgical intervention.

The scapula is a triangular-shaped bone with the glenoid fossa on the lateral surface. The bone is flat and translucent with thickened borders and ridges at the sites of the various muscle attachments. The coracoid process projects anterior, superior, and lateral from the lateral aspect of the anterior face of the scapula. Just medial to the coracoid base is the suprascapular notch, which is bridged by the transverse scapular ligament. The suprascapular nerve courses through the notch under the ligament. Surgical approaches may be directed on the lateral aspect of the coracoid, as the brachial plexus and axillary artery occur adjacent to its medial base. Along the anteromedial margin of the scapula is the origin of the serratus anterior muscle. The subscapularis muscle covers most of the anterior surface of the scapula and only the glenoid neck is devoid of muscle attachments. The long head of triceps originates on the inferior aspect of the glenoid neck, the coracobrachialis, short head of biceps, and pectoralis minor from the coracoid process, and the long head of biceps from the superior aspect of the glenoid.

On the posterior aspect of the scapula, the spine originates on the upper third and sweeps laterally

* Corresponding author.

E-mail address: plapner@ottawahospital.on.ca.
(P.C. Lapner).

and anteriorly to form the acromion. The space between the spine and acromion forms a gap, the spinoglenoid notch, around which the suprascapular nerve and artery pass to innervate the infraspinatus. The scapular spine divides the posterior scapular surface into its upper third, the supraspinatus fossa, from which the supraspinatus originates, and lower two thirds, the infraspinatus fossa, from which the infraspinatus takes its origin. The long medial border has several muscle attachments, including the levator scapulae, the rhomboideus minor, and the rhomboideus major. The lateral, oblique border sees the attachments of the latissimus dorsi, teres major, teres minor, and triceps. The deep lateral shoulder musculature is covered by the deltoid. The posterior and middle heads of the deltoid muscle originate along a broad base on the posterior rim of the spine and lateral border of the acromion, and the trapezius inserts on the superior rim of the spine. The anterior deltoid originates on the clavicle and anterior acromial rim. The acromioclavicular, glenohumeral, and sternoclavicular joints are the articulations that make up the shoulder complex. The dorsal scapular and accessory nerves travel with the superficial and deep branches of the transverse cervical artery parallel and medial to the medial border of the scapula.

Positioning of the hand in space requires the coordinated activity of the glenohumeral and scapulothoracic joints. Scapular malunion, nonunion, scarring, nerve injury, or muscle damage can limit the smooth motion of the scapula against the chest wall. This limitation in turn affects the normal scapulohumeral rhythm and can therefore affect the normal functioning of the upper limb.

Classification of scapular fractures

Certain fracture patterns are seen in the scapula and are described by anatomic area for ease of discussion. Several areas of the scapula may be involved simultaneously but fractures that involve the glenoid neck and scapular body are the most common [4–7].

Goss [8,9] described the superior shoulder suspensory complex (SSSC). In this complex, the upper limb is suspended by two struts and a ring (Fig. 1). The superior strut consists of the middle clavicle, and the scapular body and spine make up the inferior strut. The ring is made up of the lateral clavicle, acromioclavicular ligaments, acromion, coracoid process, and the coracoclavicular

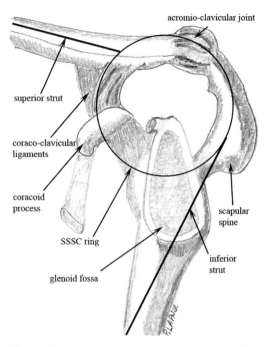

Fig. 1. The superior suspensory shoulder complex. (*Adapted from* Goss TP. Double disruptions of the superior shoulder suspensory complex. J Orthop Trauma 1993;7(2):99–106; with permission.)

ligaments. The ring is a semirigid construct, although limited motion may occur through its ligamentous components.

Simple disruptions of the ring can occur with relatively minor trauma. Because these injuries are stable, they can often be treated nonoperatively. Disruptions that occur at two sites in the ring, so called "double disruptions," create a situation in which the ring becomes potentially unstable. These can take the form of either a ring disruption with concomitant disruption of one strut, or both struts may be involved. An example of this would involve a fracture of the glenoid neck with a concomitant fracture of the middle third of the clavicle, which is analogous to a "floating shoulder." Similarly, an isolated fracture of the coracoid does not destabilize the ring. A fracture of both the clavicle and the acromion creates an unstable situation, however. Instability in this setting may be problematic for the healing of fractures and subsequent function, and may predispose to glenohumeral arthrosis [9].

Fractures of the glenoid fossa have been classified by Ideberg and colleagues [3]. These are described in further detail later in this article.

Avulsion fractures of bony prominences and stress fractures through indirect forces at the attachment of muscles or ligaments may also occur. These fractures can involve the superomedial angle of the scapula, the superior scapular border, the tip of the coracoid process, the superior aspect of the coracoid process, the acromial margin, and the inferior angle of the scapula. In isolation, most such fractures heal well with nonoperative management [10].

Clinical and radiographic evaluation

Knowledge of the history of the mechanism of injury aids in diagnosis and subsequent treatment. Injuries that involve a fall on the outstretched arm or dislocation of the shoulder can result in glenoid rim fractures. High-energy blunt trauma to the forequarter may be associated with fractures of the scapular body or glenoid neck with possible extension into the glenoid fossa. Inferiorly directed forces from above may lead to fractures of the scapular spine or acromion. Traction mechanisms can result in injuries that range from avulsion fractures of the scapular processes to major neurovascular compromise associated with brachial plexus avulsion.

Physical examination may reveal a flattened appearance of the shoulder if the fracture involves the scapular spine or acromion. The degree of ecchymosis can be less than one would expect with this degree of injury. Tenderness to palpation occurs over the site of soft tissue and bone injury. The arm is typically held in an adducted position and any attempted motion is resisted because of pain. It is important to document any associated neurologic deficits. Significant swelling in the rotator cuff can lead to muscular inhibition and the syndrome of "pseudo–cuff rupture" [11]. This injury manifests clinically as the inability to raise the arm actively, but the syndrome usually resolves in a matter of weeks.

Associated injuries occur in 80% to 95% of patients who have fractures of the scapula [4,6,7,12]. The most commonly associated lesions in decreasing order of frequency are thoracic injuries [13], lesions to the contralateral extremity, cranial lesions, and spinal lesions [1,3,7,14,15]. The overall mortality rate is between 10% and 15%, usually attributable to pulmonary sepsis or head injury [1,7]. Neurologic lesions occur commonly with glenoid rim fractures [3]. Fischer and colleagues [16] reported that 70% of patients who had brachial plexus injuries had major scapular body fractures.

A prospective series of scapular fractures demonstrated a high incidence of pneumothorax, occurring in 16 of 30 patients [17]. More than half the cases were delayed in onset, occurring 1 to 3 days following the injury. The authors advocated a follow-up chest radiograph and a high degree of clinical suspicion to make the diagnosis.

A standard radiographic series for the evaluation of scapular fractures should include a true anteroposterior (AP) view of the glenohumeral joint, an axillary view, and a scapular Y view. The true AP view allows for identification of glenohumeral joint malalignment, angulation of the glenoid neck, and fractures of the scapular body. The axillary view is useful for determination of the relationship between the humeral head and glenoid fossa, status of the acromion, and integrity of the coracoid process. The scapular Y view may demonstrate angular or rotatory displacement of the glenoid and scapular body. CT scan with three-dimensional (3-D) reconstruction is likely the most useful imaging modality for surgical planning [18]. It allows for precise determination of the degree of glenoid intra-articular displacement, angulation, and overall relationship between bone fragments in these complex fractures.

Fractures of the glenoid neck (extra-articular)

Fractures of the glenoid neck occur in metaphyseal bone. The fragment that contains the glenoid fossa typically displaces distally and anteromedially because of the weight of the arm and pull of the muscles of the proximal humerus [19,20]. If the suspensory ligaments are intact, however, the fracture may remain stable [21].

The fracture line extends from the lateral border of the scapula to the superior border, either lateral to (anatomic) or medial to (surgical) the coracoid process [19]. A third type has been described in which the fracture line extends from the inferior glenoid neck to the medial border of the scapula [22]. The exit point of the fracture line, however, has not been found useful in guiding treatment or in determining prognosis.

Although the shoulder joint is considered a universal joint, there is likely a limit to how much displacement the glenohumeral joint can accommodate before function is affected. The glenopolar angle (GPA) is the most common method of determining the degree of rotational displacement of the glenoid (Fig. 2) [23]. It is the angle formed between a line drawn between the superior and inferior poles of the glenoid, and a second line from the superior glenoid pole to the inferior angle of the scapula. A GPA of 30 to 45 degrees is considered normal, and less than 20 degrees is considered severe.

A second method of measuring the glenoid inclination involves using the medial scapular border as a reference on a true AP shoulder film [24,25]. The angle is formed between the line perpendicular to a line between the superior and inferior poles of the glenoid, and a line perpendicular to the medial scapular border (Fig. 3). Van Noort and colleagues considered 20 degrees of caudal tilt significant in their multicenter study on floating shoulders. Some difficulty may arise in determining the exact orientation of the medial scapular border line because it is not always clear on a true AP film.

If nonoperative treatment is chosen, the shoulder is immobilized for comfort. Passive exercises are initiated early and active-assisted range of

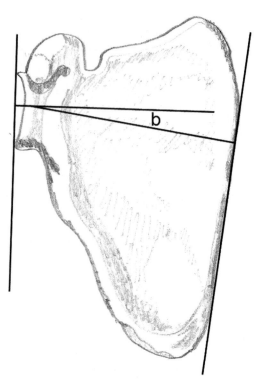

Fig. 3. The glenoid inclination. (*Data from* Gerber C. The floating shoulder: a multicentre study. J Bone Joint Surg Br 2002;84(5):776; author reply 776, with permission; and van Noort A, te Slaa RL, Marti RK, et al. The floating shoulder. A multicentre study. J Bone Joint Surg Br 2001;83(6):795–8.)

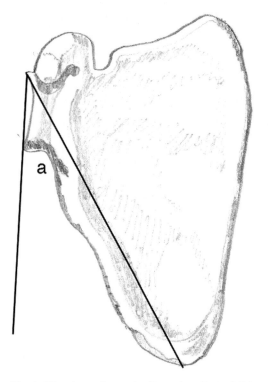

Fig. 2. The glenopolar angle. (*Data from* Bestard EA, Schvene HR. Glenoplasty in the management of recurrent shoulder dislocation. Contemp Orthop 1986;12:47.)

motion exercises are begun once there is evidence of union. Strengthening is typically begun after a full range of motion is achieved.

The decision to proceed to surgical treatment is primarily based on the degree of displacement and caudal tilt of the glenoid fragment. Ada and Miller [26] recommended surgery for fractures that were displaced more than 1 cm or angulated greater than 40 degrees. If surgery is considered, it is usually performed through a posterior approach. Screw fixation alone is not usually sufficient because of the thin quality of the scapular bone. Plate fixation with horizontally or obliquely oriented pelvic reconstruction or mini-fragment plates with multiple screws is therefore usually necessary to obtain stability (Fig. 4) [27]. Pendulum exercises may be initiated as soon as pain allows, but active-assisted motion is delayed until union occurs.

The outcomes of studies in which patients were treated nonoperatively for less severely displaced

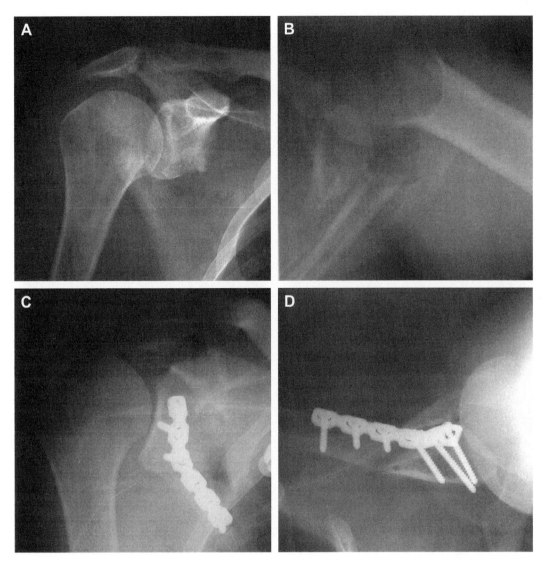

Fig. 4. Glenoid neck fracture with anterior and medial displacement. (*A*) AP radiograph showing anteriorly displacement fracture with medialization. (*B*) Axillary view. (*C*) Postoperative true AP film demonstrating reduction of the glenoid neck with pelvic reconstruction plate. (*D*) Postoperative axillary view (*Courtesy of* Allan Liew, MD, Ottawa, Ontario, Canada.)

fractures have generally been favorable. Pace and colleagues [28] studied 9 patients who had sustained a fracture of the neck of the scapula and were treated nonsurgically. Overall satisfaction levels were high at 90%, but all patients had some degree of activity-related pain. Pain was correlated with MRI evidence of subacromial impingement and minor cuff tendinopathy. The outcome of nonoperative treatment in a series of 13 patients who had glenoid neck fractures was reported by van Noort and van Kampen [29]. The mean Constant score was 90 in the series

and no correlation was found between functional outcome and malunion from medial glenoid neck displacement.

Ada and Miller [26] reported on 16 patients who had displaced glenoid neck fractures treated nonsurgically. Outcomes were not universally good: 50% had subacromial and night pain, 40% had weakness with exertion, and 20% had a decrease in range of motion. Eight patients were treated operatively with open reduction through a posterior approach. The outcomes for this latter group were better, with no pain and what they described as 85% glenohumeral motion. Based on these findings, the authors recommended that operative intervention be considered if the glenoid fragment is angulated greater than 40 degrees or has more than 1 cm of medial displacement. These indications have been supported by other authors [19,30].

Romero and colleagues [21] investigated the effect of glenoid neck rotational angulation on functional outcome. Nineteen patients were assessed for the degree of rotational misalignment of the glenoid by determining the GPA on a true AP film. Six patients had a GPA of less than 20 degrees. Of the 7 patients who had moderate or severe pain, 5 had a GPA less than 20 degrees, compared with 1 of 12 who had a GPA greater than 20 degrees. Among 5 patients who had moderately or severely impaired activities of daily living, 4 had a GPA less than 20 degrees, compared with 14 patients who had mild or no impairment of whom only 2 had a GPA less than 20 degrees.

The correlation between GPA and functional outcome as measured by the Constant score was studied by Bozkurt and colleagues [31]. The authors found a high positive correlation ($r = 0.891$) between the GPA and functional outcome in 18 patients who had glenoid neck fractures.

The outcomes of displaced, surgically treated glenoid neck fractures were reported by Khallaf and colleagues [32]. Fourteen patients were treated with open reduction and internal fixation (ORIF) of the glenoid neck, and most had associated minimally displaced acromial, spine, and scapular body fractures. At an average follow-up of 20 months, 12 patients had an excellent clinical result and 2 had a good result as measured by the University of California, Los Angeles (UCLA) score.

No studies have directly compared the outcomes of operative with nonoperative treatment. A recent meta-analysis indicated that no conclusion on operative versus nonoperative treatment can be drawn from a review of the literature on scapular neck and body fractures, because of low numbers of patients treated operatively, variability between studies, nonvalidated outcome measures, high incidence of additional associated injuries, and methodologic limitations [33]. The authors' preferred method of treatment is to consider surgical intervention if fracture displacement is greater than 1 cm or if significant caudal angulation of the glenoid fragment (GPA < 20 degrees) occurs. The

posterior approach is used for surgical exposure, and 3.5 mm pelvic reconstruction plates are contoured for optimal fixation.

Fractures of the glenoid (intra-articular)

Fractures of the glenoid cavity are intra-articular fractures that can lead to shoulder instability or glenohumeral arthrosis. As such, displaced fractures of the glenoid fossa have the poorest prognosis of all scapular injuries without operative intervention and therefore present a special challenge for the surgeon [34].

Fractures of the glenoid rim are distinct from small bone lesions that occur during shoulder dislocation in which a small avulsion fracture occurs at the site of capsulolabral attachment [35]. Fractures of the glenoid fossa occur when violent force is applied laterally that directs the humeral head against the glenoid fossa [4]. A transverse fracture occurs, which then propagates in one of various directions depending on the direction of the force.

Ideberg and colleagues [3] proposed a classification system that included fractures of the glenoid rim and fossa, based on a review of 300 fractures of the glenoid cavity (Fig. 5): type I, fractures of the glenoid rim; type IA, anterior; and type IB, posterior; type II, transverse fractures through the glenoid fossa with an inferior glenoid fragment that displaces with the humeral head; type III, transverse fracture that exits in the mid-superior scapula and often associated with acromioclavicular fracture or dislocation; type IV, transverse fracture that extends to the medial scapular border; and type V, similar to type IV with extension of a secondary fracture line to the lateral scapular border resulting in the formation of a separate inferior glenoid fragment. Goss [35] included a sixth type, involving severe comminution of the glenoid cavity.

Nonoperative treatment is indicated for minimally displaced fractures of the glenoid rim or fossa. Immobilization in a sling and swathe is used for relief of pain. Early progressive range-of-motion exercises are initiated as soon as the pain subsides. Close radiographic follow-up is recommended and union usually occurs by 6 weeks. Functional use of the shoulder for activities of daily living is allowed and an active range-of-motion program is initiated. Resistive strengthening exercises are begun once range of motion is restored.

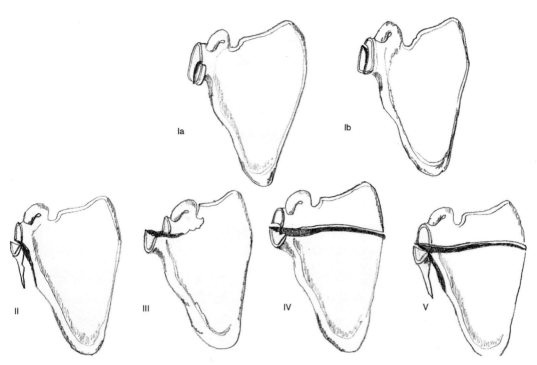

Fig. 5. The Ideberg classification of glenoid fossa fractures. (*Data from* Ideberg R, Grevsten S, Larsson S. Epidemiology of scapular fractures. Incidence and classification of 338 fractures. Acta Orthop Scand 1995;66(5):395–7.)

Close radiographic follow-up is recommended if the nonoperative approach is taken. Recurrent instability of the shoulder can occur following reduction and a persistent, chronic dislocation can result, especially in older patients [36].

General indications for surgery in fractures of the fossa include a step of 5 mm at the articular surface, or a significant gap with displacement of the inferior fragment that results in subluxation of the humeral head [35].

The two main surgical approaches for fixation of glenoid fractures are the deltopectoral approach and the posterior approach. The anterior deltopectoral approach involves division of the subscapularis tendon 1.5 cm medial to the intertubercular groove. The tenotomy is carried inferiorly to the level of the anterior circumflex humeral vessels. Care is taken to protect the vessels and the axillary nerve at the inferior border of the subscapularis tendon. The subscapularis is tagged and reflected medially as it is separated from the underlying capsule. A capsulotomy is performed and insertion of a humeral head retractor permits visualization to the entire glenoid fossa with wide access to the anterior glenoid rim.

In the posterior approach, the deltoid fibers may be divided, and the interval between infraspinatus and teres minor is developed exposing the posterior neck and capsule. Alternatively, the deltoid can be detached from the spine, and the infraspinatus is elevated from its fossa and retracted superiorly with inferior retraction on teres minor. The infraspinatus is divided 1.5 cm medial to its insertion on the greater tuberosity and along its superior and inferior borders. A posterior capsulotomy and retraction of the humeral head allow access to the entire glenoid cavity with wide access to the posterior glenoid rim. If exposure of the superior glenoid is required, the incision is extended superiorly. The trapezius is elevated from the clavicle, and the supraspinatus fibers are split for exposure of the superior glenoid and coracoid process. Excision of the distal clavicle may be necessary to improve exposure and for the insertion of internal fixation [34].

The main indication for operative intervention for type I fractures is fracture displacement sufficient enough to result in subluxation of the humeral head. This injury is most likely to occur with anterior rim fractures involving one fourth of the articular surface and 10 mm displacement anteriorly, or one third of the articular surface posteriorly [37]. Ideberg and colleagues' [3] indication for operative intervention was persistent subluxation, or recurrent instability following closed reduction. Of 130 patients in their report, 125 had a satisfactory outcome. Eleven patients in the series were treated surgically for the aforementioned indication, and 5 had a satisfactory result.

The anterior approach is well suited for access to anterior glenoid rim and coracoid fractures.

Larger fragments can be addressed with interfragmentary compression using lag-screw technique with small-fragment cortical screws to the glenoid neck (Fig. 6). Smaller or multi-fragmentary fractures not amenable to internal fixation should be excised. The defect can be grafted with a tri-cortical iliac crest bone graft [12,19,38]. A Latarjet-type coracoid transfer may also be used, depending on the preference of the surgeon. Reattachment of the labrum to the remaining glenoid rim with no bony reconstruction likely

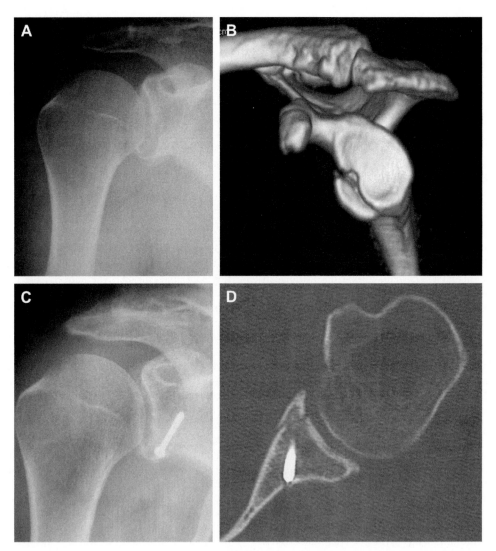

Fig. 6. Anterior glenoid fracture. (*A*) Preoperative plain film showing displaced glenoid lip fracture. (*B*) Preoperative 3-D CT scan. (*C*) Postoperative axillary view with anterior screw fixation. (*D*) Postoperative axial CT demonstrating anatomic reduction.

does not confer the same degree of stability [39,40]. The surgical principles are identical for posterior glenoid rim fractures, for which the posterior approach is used.

Type II fractures can occur in either transverse or oblique orientation and result in an inferior glenoid fragment. A 5-mm intra-articular step or inferior subluxation of the humeral head can occur with displacement and should lead the surgeon to consider ORIF [12,38]. A posterior approach is best suited for exposure. A superiorly directed interfragmentary screw or a buttress plate applied to the posterior glenoid neck provides optimal fixation [19,38].

Type III fractures involve the upper third of the glenoid fossa and include the coracoid process. ORIF should be considered for an intra-articular step of 5 mm [9]. An anterior approach combined with a superior approach for insertion of an inferiorly directed screw may be considered [10]. If a superior approach is chosen, the supraspinatus fibers are split for exposure of the superior glenoid. The lateral clavicle may be excised to allow for insertion of the screws. Reduction and fixation of associated injuries in the superior shoulder suspensor complex may result in improvement in fracture alignment and improved stability. Five of Ideberg's 17 cases had a poor result, which was attributed to associated injuries.

Type IV fractures extend to the medial border of the scapula. As in type III, open reduction should be considered if a significant intra-articular step or gap occurs, particularly if the superior fragment is displaced laterally [12,35]. As with type III fractures, a posterosuperior approach is used with an inferiorly directed screw from the superior scapular neck to the inferior neck.

Type V fractures are a combination of the fracture patterns seen in type II and IV. Indications for surgery are similar to those described for those two fractures, respectively. Nonoperative treatment may be considered if the head is well centered [10,12,35].

Operative treatment of type VI fractures is generally contraindicated, because surgical dissection of the already compromised soft tissue envelope may lead to a more deleterious result. Some authors have suggested that immobilization of the arm in a shoulder spica or similar splint, in a position that maximizes articular surface congruity, may be beneficial. After 2 weeks, a sling and swathe may be used with progressive functional use and range-of-motion exercises as the symptoms allow. Other injuries to the SSSC may be addressed surgically because this may improve the alignment of the comminuted glenoid fossa fracture [19,35].

Arthroscopy is increasingly being used in the evaluation and treatment of glenoid fractures. The procedure is technically demanding, however, and few reports in the literature have documented its effectiveness [41,42]. The technique allows for good visualization of all aspects of the glenohumeral articulation and the benefit of leaving the anterior or posterior musculotendinous units intact as compared with an open approach. Reduction may be easier to gauge with this technique if no communion is present. Percutaneously placed 3.0- or 3.5-mm cannulated screws are ideal for fracture fixation [43]. A suture fixation technique has also been described that is analogous to the technique for arthroscopic Bankart repair described by Casperi and colleagues [41,44].

Adam and colleagues [45] reported on the operative treatment of 10 patients who had displaced glenoid fractures. All fractures were united by 6 to 8 weeks. At a minimum of 18 months' follow-up, 8 of 10 patients had good or excellent functional results. Schandelmaier and colleagues [46] reported on 22 patients treated with ORIF for displacement glenoid fractures, with a minimum of 5-year follow-up. The mean Constant score was 79, and 4 patients had a score less than 50. Two of the patients who had poor results had deep infections, and the other 2 had complete brachial plexus palsy. The authors concluded that ORIF yielded good or excellent results in patients whose postoperative course was free of complications.

Hardegger and colleagues [19] reported on 12 patients who underwent ORIF of the glenoid. They recommended operative intervention for incongruent fractures of the glenoid, but the outcome of these particular patients was not reported separately from the larger series. Kavanagh and colleagues [47] reported on 9 patients treated surgically for glenoid fractures through a posterior approach with a mean follow-up of 4 years. Eight patients had few or no symptoms and full range of motion. No patient developed joint arthrosis. The patients were satisfied with the outcome but no validated outcome score was used. Leung and colleagues [48] reported on a series of 14 patients treated with ORIF. At a follow-up of 30.5 months, all had achieved good results using the Rowe scoring system. The authors advocated a posterior approach in all glenoid fractures except type III, for which an anterior approach was used.

Mayo and colleagues [34] reported on 27 patients who underwent ORIF of glenoid fossa fractures with a mean follow-up of 43 months. Anatomic reduction was possible in 89% of cases. Functional evaluation revealed a good or excellent outcome in 82%, and a fair or poor outcome in 18%. The poorer outcomes were attributed to associated neurologic and acromioclavicular joint trauma.

Scapular body fractures

Fractures to the scapular body may result from direct trauma, most commonly from a fall or motor vehicle collision, or from seizures that occur secondary to electric shock [49–51]. Nonoperative treatment of scapular fractures usually results in a favorable outcome, and nonunion is rare. The extensive soft tissue envelope that surrounds the scapula results in a high rate of union, and normal bony anatomy is not necessary for normal shoulder function [10]. Fractures that heal in a displaced position may result in a grating sensation at the scapulothoracic interface but that usually does not interfere with function [26]. Shoulder immobilization and ice are used initially for comfort. Pendulum exercises and progressive range of motion are begun within 1 week of injury.

Ogawa and Yoshida [51] reported on 24 fractures of the superior border of the scapula. All were associated with other injuries, including glenoid fossa fractures in 9 patients. Other associated injuries included fractures of the coracoid, lateral clavicle, spine, and dislocations of the acromioclavicular joint. Of 18 patients treated at their institution, 8 were treated surgically; all operations were directed at the associated injuries and not at the scapular body fractures. All patients achieved excellent results according the Neer's criteria at an average 2-year follow-up.

Not all reports on the nonoperative treatment of scapula fractures have shown favorable results. Nordqvist and Petersson [30] reported on 41 fractures of the scapular body as part of a larger series. Outcome was based on patient satisfaction and range of motion. Of 34 fractures that were displaced less than 10 mm, 29 had a good result. In contrast, of 7 fractures displaced greater than 10 mm, only 3 had a good result.

A special consideration in the surgical treatment of scapular body fractures is the site and positioning of internal fixation. The optimal sites of fixation based on scapular thickness were investigated by Burke and colleagues [52]. Eighteen cadaver scapulae were studied: the glenoid fossa (25 mm), lateral scapular border (9.7 mm), and scapular spine (8.3 mm) were the sites of greatest thickness and thus optimal sites for internal fixation.

The author's preferred method of treatment is to determine the degree of scapular body fracture displacement with the aid of two-dimensional and 3-D CT scan reconstructions. If significant displacement (>10 mm) occurs at the spine or lateral border, then internal fixation is considered. Most fractures, however, can be managed nonoperatively.

The floating shoulder

The term "floating shoulder" was originally used to describe a fracture of the clavicle and ipsilateral glenoid neck, effectively dissociating the upper extremity from the axial skeleton. More recently, it has been used to designate a combination of fractures that occur in the scapular neck, spine, coracoid process, acromion, or clavicle. We define the term to describe a specific combination of fractures involving both the clavicle and glenoid neck [53]. The concepts that guide treatment and the roles that the coracoclavicular, acromioclavicular, and coracoacromial ligaments play in stabilizing these injuries are evolving. A thorough understanding of the pathoanatomy and mechanisms that stabilize the shoulder girdle is necessary if an effective treatment plan is to be formulated.

Goss [9] warned that if two points of disruption occur within the superior shoulder suspensory complex, the ring becomes unstable. This disruption may occur in the setting of two fractures that occur within the ring, or a fracture that occurs in combination with a disruption of one of the ligamentous components. This instability may in turn lead to delayed or nonunion, malunion, weakness, or late glenohumeral arthrosis, and thus some authors have advocated surgical intervention in this setting [8,20].

Williams and colleagues [54], however, reported on biomechanical data that suggested that fractures of the glenoid neck and clavicle are not inherently unstable. The authors observed that disruption of the acromioclavicular and coracoclavicular ligaments are required for loss of stability to occur at the glenoid neck.

Several reports on the nonoperative treatment of floating shoulder injuries have appeared in the literature. Not knowing the status of the suspensory shoulder ligaments makes it difficult to determine the exact role that they play in the context of fracture displacement, however.

Edwards and colleagues [53] reported on the nonoperative treatment of 20 patients who had ipsilateral clavicle and scapular fractures. Eleven clavicle fractures were displaced greater than 10 mm, and five scapular fractures were displaced greater than 5 mm. Ninety-five percent of fractures healed without incident. At a mean follow-up of 28 months, the average Rowe score was 95 and the mean Constant score was 96. No weakness was found compared with the contralateral side. The authors concluded that nonoperative treatment may be considered in the management of these injuries within the range of displacement cited earlier. The results of 16 patients who had scapular neck and clavicle fractures treated nonoperatively were reported by Ramos and colleagues [55]. A success rate of 92% was found at 7.5-year follow-up. All but 1 patient had minimal fracture displacement.

Surgical stabilization of one disruption may sufficiently stabilize the ring to avoid these complications. Herscovici and colleagues [20] reported on seven patients who had glenoid neck fractures with ipsilateral mid-shaft clavicle fractures. All patients were treated with ORIF of the clavicle fractures. All patients achieved an excellent functional result with no residual deformity at 48.5-month follow-up; this was in contrast to two other patients in the series who were treated nonoperatively. Both had shoulder drooping and decreased range of motion. Hashiguchi and Ito [56] reported on five patients who had minimally displaced fractures of the scapular neck and ipsilateral clavicle fractures. The scapula neck fracture included the coracoid in all cases. Operative fixation was undertaken for the clavicle fractures alone either with plates and screws or with K-wires. The authors reported union in all cases and a UCLA score of 34.2 at a mean follow-up of 57.4 months.

Several studies investigated the outcomes of operative versus nonoperative intervention. van Noort and colleagues [25] investigated 35 patients in a multicenter study who had concomitant scapular and clavicle fractures. The mean Constant score was 76 for the 28 patients treated nonsurgically and 76 for the 7 patients treated operatively at a mean follow-up of 35 months. The 6 patients who had untreated caudal "dislocation" of the glenoid had a Constant score of 42, and the 22 patients who did not have this finding had a score of 85. The authors concluded that this injury is not inherently unstable, but that the outcome depends on the adequacy of reduction of the glenoid. Three patients in the series had persistent malunion of the glenoid neck fractures despite anatomic reduction and fixation of the clavicle fractures. Egol and colleagues [57] reported on a series of 19 patients who had ipsilateral glenoid neck and clavicular or acromioclavicular joint disruption. Twelve patients were treated nonoperatively and the remainder were treated with operative fixation of both injuries. At a mean follow-up of 53 months, no significant differences between groups were found with the American Shoulder and Elbow Surgeons shoulder scale, the Disabilities of the Arm, Shoulder, and Hand, or with the Short Form-36. Strength in internal and external rotation was greater in the nonoperatively treated group. The only parameter that favored the operatively treated group was range of motion in forward elevation. Labler and colleagues [58] reported on 17 patients who had floating shoulder injuries. Eight patients were treated nonoperatively, and 9 were treated with ORIF of either one or both injuries. Five patients in each group demonstrated good to excellent functional results. The decision to operate was left to the surgeons' discretion and was based on the degree of displacement of the injuries and the presence of concomitant injuries. Oh and colleagues [59] reviewed 13 cases who had fractures of glenoid neck and clavicle with a mean follow-up of 1 year. Three patients were treated nonsurgically, 5 had fixation of the clavicle alone, and 5 had fixation of the clavicle and scapula. Functional assessment by the Rowe score was 88 in patients treated surgically compared with 77 in patients treated without surgery. The authors recommended surgical treatment of double disruptions of the superior shoulder suspensory complex when both struts are involved.

Leung and Lam [60] reported on a 15 cases of glenoid neck fractures associated with fractures of the clavicle. They recommended ORIF of both the clavicle and glenoid fractures. Union occurred by 8 weeks in all cases. At a mean follow-up of 25 months, the functional outcome as measured by the Rowe score was good or excellent in all but one patient. Several complications occurred, however: one patient developed a pneumothorax, one required plate removal because of irritation, and five had pain attributed to irritation of the plate.

It is the opinion of some authors that glenoid neck fractures displace because of the lateralization of the scapular body and not purely because of the medialization of the glenoid fracture fragment secondary to the force applied from the rotator cuff [61,62]. The mobility of the scapular body, the weight of the arm, and the pull of the long head of triceps, biceps, and rotator cuff may allow this to occur. Reduction in this setting would involve medialization of the scapular body fragment with subsequent reduction of the glenoid neck fragment.

In conclusion, the evidence to direct the treatment of floating shoulder injuries is not clear. Because of the rarity of the injury, studies on the subject are limited to retrospective case series. The studies that have attempted to provide a comparison of outcomes for surgical versus nonoperative treatment had several confounding variables [20,29,57–59]. The biomechanical evidence suggests that dual fractures of the glenoid neck and clavicle are not necessary unstable in the absence of ligamentous disruption [54]. It is therefore unlikely that stabilization of the clavicle alone is necessary in all cases. It is the authors' opinion that persistent caudal angulation of the glenoid should lead the surgeon to consider operative intervention. If caudal angulation of the glenoid fragment persists after stabilization of the clavicle, reduction and fixation of the glenoid should be considered, within the context of the fracture pattern and the patient's general status.

Scapulothoracic dissociations

A review of scapular injuries would be incomplete without a discussion of traumatic scapulothoracic dissociation (SD). In contrast to most scapular body fractures resulting from significant blunt force, these injuries most commonly occur from a severe traction mechanism. More than 50% of reported injuries occur in motorcycle accidents, but other motor vehicle accidents, pedestrian accidents, falls from heights, and other high-energy mechanisms can lead to this injury. Oreck and colleagues [63] originally described this injury as a complete disruption of the scapulothoracic articulation with lateral scapular displacement and intact skin. Some surgeons have termed the injury an internal forequarter amputation in severe cases.

In SD, the scapular body and arm are lateralized and all or most of the muscular and ligamentous structures are injured, including the rhomboids, levator scapulae, trapezius, latissimus dorsi, pectoralis muscles, and others. A dislocation of the sternoclavicular joint, acromioclavicular joint, or most commonly a distracted midshaft clavicle fracture usually accompanies the soft tissue injury (Fig. 7). Other associated bony injuries of the scapular body, humerus, or upper extremity are common. With the muscular, ligamentous, and bony injury, the scapula and arm are essentially torn away from the thorax. Although there is likely a spectrum of injury, most case series are based on the most severe injuries. In these series, vascular injuries (88%) and neurologic deficits (94%) in the affected arm are extremely common [64]. Treatment is mainly directed at the vascular and neurologic injuries of the arm [65].

Because this injury involves extreme force, associated visceral injuries are common. In one review, 86% of patients had significant associated injuries, including cranial, thoracic, abdominal, and other major orthopedic fractures [64]. The mortality rate was 11% among these patients. The first step in assessment of these severely injured patients often includes the full trauma service. Resuscitation is begun and the severe concomitant injuries are dealt with on an emergent

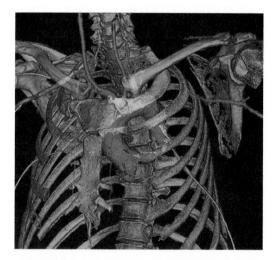

Fig. 7. CT Reconstruction of a patient who had SD. Note sternoclavicular dislocation, significant lateralization of the scapula, and the subclavian artery injury. (*From* Scapulothoracic dissociation with subclavian artery dissection following a severe motorbike accident. Eur J Cardiothorac Surg 2006;30(4):671; with permission.)

basis. Surprisingly, the severity of other injuries can draw attention away from the arm and the SD can be missed [66].

Assessment

On inspection of the arm, massive soft tissue swelling and hematoma formation are present but may not always be readily apparent. Gross instability of the proximal extremity and pain with palpation or motion may be present. Signs of vascular compromise, including delayed capillary refill, distal extremity discoloration, coldness, or lack of pulses, should be sought. Doppler ultrasound can be helpful to assess pulses and pulse pressures in a fashion similar to performing an ankle-brachial index. A full neurologic examination of all dermatomes, myotomes, and peripheral nerves should be performed and the location of any neurologic deficit identified. Horner syndrome (miosis, ptosis, anhydrosis, enophthalmos) would suggest a preganglionic nerve injury at the level of T1. Diaphragm function should be evaluated.

Radiographs are based on clinical assessment but the affected extremity should be screened for associated fractures. The classic finding of SD is scapular lateralization on chest radiograph. By measuring the distance between the thoracic spinous processes and the medial scapular border bilaterally, the scapular index can be determined. In a review of 25 patients who had this condition, the average scapular index was 1.29 [67]. A higher degree of lateralization may carry an increased risk for extensive injury. The scapular index is helpful in confirming the diagnosis but may not be positive in every case. Angiogram is necessary if there is any concern for vascular injury. MRI of the neck and shoulder may be helpful to help assess the nerve and soft tissue injury. Electromyogram is used in the nonacute phase to follow nerve recovery.

Treatment

A classification system described by Damschen and revised by Zelle can help guide the treatment of this condition (Table 1) [64,67]. In type 1 injuries, the degree of muscular and bony injury is assessed, and treatment is directed on an individual basis. Initial treatment commonly involves sling immobilization and analgesic medication. Physiotherapy is instituted as soon as the pain symptoms allow. Displaced clavicle fractures may benefit from early surgery in some cases [68].

Table 1
Classification of scapulothoracic dissociation

Type	Clinical findings
Type 1	Isolated MSK injury
Type 2A	MSK injury with vascular injury
Type 2B	MSK injury with incomplete neurologic injury
Type 3	MSK injury with incomplete neurologic injury and vascular injury
Type 4	MSK injury with complete brachial plexus avulsion

Abbreviation: MSK, musculoskeletal.

In type 2A injuries, assessment of the vascular injury should include an angiogram and a vascular surgery consultation is required. In patients who show signs of hemodynamic instability in whom the source of blood loss is considered to be the SD, emergent surgery should be performed. Surgical options include arterial repair, bypass, or simply tying off the subclavian artery. The anastomotic network surrounding the shoulder is abundant and distal perfusion is often present despite a subclavian artery injury [69]. Venous bleeding can be tied off or packed.

Hemodynamic stability may be maintained in the setting of a subclavian or axillary artery avulsion. The decision to operate follows a similar algorithm. If ischemia is present in the distal limb, emergent surgery to restore perfusion is required. If the arm remains well perfused, the decision to perform surgery can be made on a case-by-case basis. In one small series, six limbs were treated with reperfusion and five limbs were treated conservatively; surgery showed no advantage [70]. Late hemorrhage from an unrepaired subclavian artery has been documented; patients should be monitored carefully if nonoperative treatment is chosen [64].

In types 2B, 3, and 4 injuries, treatment is based on several factors. In cases in which the vascular injury mandates surgery, brachial plexus exploration can be considered in the acute phase once the patient is stable. Early repair, either by direct repair or nerve grafting, is often less complex than delayed reconstruction. If upper root avulsion has occurred, a delayed neurotization or tendon transfer may be considered. In cases of complete brachial plexus avulsion, early above-elbow amputation should be considered.

If the vascular injury does not mandate early surgery, treatment of any plexus injury is initially nonoperative. Nerve function is assessed and all deficits are documented. Although it is not possible to discuss all options for partial brachial plexus injuries in this article, referral to an expert may be warranted. Complete brachial plexus palsy, with no signs of function on a delayed basis, carries a poor prognosis for any recovery and amputation of the flail arm should be considered [67]. Preoperative consultation and planning for prosthetic replacement is important in this setting.

Outcome

The outcome of these devastating injuries is generally poor, but most closely correlates with nerve function [67]. In one series, 21% had early amputation, 52% of patients had a flail arm, and the remaining had variable function [64]. In many cases, patients refuse amputation and choose to live with the flail arm on a long-term basis.

Summary

Scapular fractures occur in the setting of high-energy trauma. They are often accompanied by potentially life-threatening injuries that frequently involve the thorax, spine, and head. Because initial treatment is usually directed at these concomitant injuries, a high index of suspicion is required to detect scapular involvement. Most fractures that involve the scapula may be treated nonoperatively and a good outcome can be expected. Specific fracture patterns, however, should alert the surgeon that operative intervention may improve outcome. The concepts that guide operative management are continuing to evolve, and future prospective studies will certainly improve our understanding of these complex injuries.

Acknowledgment

We thank Ms. Kimberly Bell for her assistance in the preparation of this manuscript.

References

[1] Thompson DA, Flynn TC, Miller PW, et al. The significance of scapular fractures. J Trauma 1985; 25(10):974–7.

[2] Rowe CR. Fractures of the scapula. Surg Clin North Am 1963;43:1565–71.

[3] Ideberg R, Grevsten S, Larsson S. Epidemiology of scapular fractures. Incidence and classification of 338 fractures. Acta Orthop Scand 1995;66(5):395–7.

[4] McGahan JP, Rab GT, Dublin A. Fractures of the scapula. J Trauma 1980;20(10):880–3.

[5] Wilber MC, Evans EB. Fractures of the scapula. An analysis of forty cases and a review of the literature. J Bone Joint Surg Am 1977;59(3):358–62.

[6] Imatani RJ. Fractures of the scapula: a review of 53 fractures. J Trauma 1975;15(6):473–8.

[7] Armstrong CP, Van der Spuy J. The fractured scapula: importance and management based on a series of 62 patients. Injury 1984;15(5):324–9.

[8] Goss TP. Double disruptions of the superior shoulder suspensory complex. J Orthop Trauma 1993; 7(2):99–106.

[9] Goss TP. Scapular fractures and dislocations: diagnosis and treatment. J Am Acad Orthop Surg 1995;3(1):22–33.

[10] Butters KP. The scapula. In: Rockwood CA, Matsen FA III, editors. The shoulder. Philadelphia: WB Saunders; 1998. p. 391–427.

[11] Neviaser JS. Traumatic lesions; injuries in and about the shoulder joint. Instr Course Lect 1956;13: 187–216.

[12] Guttentag IJ, Rechtine GR. Fractures of the scapula. A review of the literature. Orthop Rev 1988; 17(2):147–58.

[13] Veysi VT, Mittal R, Agarwal S, et al. Multiple trauma and scapula fractures: so what? J Trauma 2003;55(6):1145–7.

[14] McGinnis M, Denton JR. Fractures of the scapula: a retrospective study of 40 fractured scapulae. J Trauma 1989;29(11):1488–93.

[15] Weening B, Walton C, Cole PA, et al. Lower mortality in patients with scapular fractures. J Trauma 2005;59(6):1477–81.

[16] Fischer RP, Flynn TC, Miller PW, et al. Scapular fractures and associated major ipsilateral upper torso injuries. Current Concepts in Trauma Care 1985;1:14–6.

[17] McLennen JG, Ungersma J. Pneumothorax complicating fractures of the scapula. J Bone Joint Surg Am 1982;64:598–9.

[18] Tadros AM, Lunsjo K, Czechowski J, et al. Usefulness of different imaging modalities in the assessment of scapular fractures caused by blunt trauma. Acta Radiol 2007;48(1):71–5.

[19] Hardegger FH, Simpson LA, Weber BG. The operative treatment of scapular fractures. J Bone Joint Surg Br 1984;66(5):725–31.

[20] Herscovici D Jr, Fiennes AG, Allgower M, et al. The floating shoulder: ipsilateral clavicle and scapular neck fractures. J Bone Joint Surg Br 1992;74(3): 362–4.

[21] Romero J, Schai P, Imhoff AB. Scapular neck fracture—the influence of permanent malalignment of the glenoid neck on clinical outcome. Arch Orthop Trauma Surg 2001;121(6):313–6.

[22] Miller ME, Ada JR. Fractures of the scapula, clavicle, and glenoid. In: Browner BD, Jupiter JB, Levine AM, editors. Skeletal trauma: fractures,

dislocations, ligamentous injuries, vol. 2Philadelphia: WB Saunders; 1992. p. 1291–310.

[23] Bestard EA, Schvene HR. Glenoplasty in the management of recurrent shoulder dislocation. Contemp Orthop 1986;12:47.

[24] Gerber C. The floating shoulder: a multicentre study. J Bone Joint Surg Br 2002;84(5):776 [author reply: 776].

[25] van Noort A, te Slaa RL, Marti RK, et al. The floating shoulder. A multicentre study. J Bone Joint Surg Br 2001;83(6):795–8.

[26] Ada JR, Miller ME. Scapular fractures. Analysis of 113 cases. Clin Orthop Relat Res 1991;269:174–80.

[27] de Beer JF, Berghs BM, van Rooyen KS, et al. Displaced scapular neck fracture: a case report. J Shoulder Elbow Surg 2004;13(1):123–5.

[28] Pace AM, Stuart R, Brownlow H. Outcome of glenoid neck fractures. J Shoulder Elbow Surg 2005; 14(6):585–90.

[29] van Noort A, van Kampen A. Fractures of the scapula surgical neck: outcome after conservative treatment in 13 cases. Arch Orthop Trauma Surg 2005; 125(10):696–700.

[30] Nordqvist A, Petersson C. Fracture of the body, neck, or spine of the scapula. A long-term follow-up study. Clin Orthop Relat Res 1992;283:139–44.

[31] Bozkurt M, Can F, Kirdemir V, et al. Conservative treatment of scapular neck fracture: the effect of stability and glenopolar angle on clinical outcome. Injury 2005;36(10):1176–81.

[32] Khallaf F, Mikami A, Al-Akkad M. The use of surgery in displaced scapular neck fractures. Med Princ Pract 2006;15(6):443–8.

[33] Zlowodzki M, Bhandari M, Zelle BA, et al. Treatment of scapula fractures: systematic review of 520 fractures in 22 case series. J Orthop Trauma 2006; 20(3):230–3.

[34] Mayo KA, Benirschke SK, Mast JW. Displaced fractures of the glenoid fossa. Results of open reduction and internal fixation. Clin Orthop Relat Res 1998;347:122–30.

[35] Goss TP. Fractures of the glenoid cavity. J Bone Joint Surg Am 1992;74(2):299–305.

[36] Kummel BM. Fractures of the glenoid causing chronic dislocation of the shoulder. Clin Orthop Relat Res 1970;69:189–91.

[37] Depalma AF. Surgery of the shoulder. 3rd edition. Philadelphia: JB Lippincott; 1983. p. 3667.

[38] Aulicino PL, Reinert C, Kornberg M, et al. Displaced intra-articular glenoid fractures treated by open reduction and internal fixation. J Trauma 1986;26(12):1137–41.

[39] Burkhart SS, De Beer JF, Barth JR, et al. Results of modified Latarjet reconstruction in patients with anteroinferior instability and significant bone loss. Arthroscopy 2007;23(10):1033–41.

[40] Burkhart SS, De Beer JF. Traumatic glenohumeral bone defects and their relationship to failure of arthroscopic Bankart repairs: significance of the inverted-pear glenoid and the humeral engaging Hill-Sachs lesion. Arthroscopy 2000;16(7):677–94.

[41] Bauer T, Abadie O, Hardy P. Arthroscopic treatment of glenoid fractures. Arthroscopy 2006;22(5): 569 e1–6.

[42] Papagelopoulos PJ, Koundis GL, Kateros KT, et al. Fractures of the glenoid cavity: assessment and management. Orthopedics 1999;22(10):956–61.

[43] Cameron SE. Arthroscopic reduction and internal fixation of an anterior glenoid fracture. Arthroscopy 1998;14(7):743–6.

[44] Casperi R, Saume F. Arthroscopic reconstruction of the shoulder: the Bankart repair. In: McGinty J, editor. Operative arthroscopy. New York: Raven; 1997. p. 695–707.

[45] Adam FF. Surgical treatment of displaced fractures of the glenoid cavity. Int Orthop 2002;26(3):150–3.

[46] Schandelmaier P, Blauth M, Schneider C, et al. Fractures of the glenoid treated by operation. A 5- to 23-year follow-up of 22 cases. J Bone Joint Surg Br 2002;84(2):173–7.

[47] Kavanagh BF, Bradway JK, Cofield RH. Open reduction and internal fixation of displaced intra-articular fractures of the glenoid fossa. J Bone Joint Surg Am 1993;75(4):479–84.

[48] Leung KS, Lam TP, Poon KM. Operative treatment of displaced intra-articular glenoid fractures. Injury 1993;24(5):324–8.

[49] Kotak BP, Haddo O, Iqbal M, et al. Bilateral scapular fractures after electrocution. J R Soc Med 2000; 93(3):143–4.

[50] Rana M, Banerjee R. Scapular fracture after electric shock. Ann R Coll Surg Engl 2006;88(2):3–4.

[51] Ogawa K, Yoshida A. Fracture of the superior border of the scapula. Int Orthop 1997;21(6):371–3.

[52] Burke CS, Roberts CS, Nyland JA, et al. Scapular thickness—implications for fracture fixation. J Shoulder Elbow Surg 2006;15(5):645–8.

[53] Edwards SG, Whittle AP, Wood GW 2nd. Nonoperative treatment of ipsilateral fractures of the scapula and clavicle. J Bone Joint Surg Am 2000;82(6): 774–80.

[54] Williams GR Jr, Naranja J, Klimkiewicz J, et al. The floating shoulder: a biomechanical basis for classification and management. J Bone Joint Surg Am 2001;83-A(8):1182–7.

[55] Ramos L, Mencia R, Alonso A, et al. Conservative treatment of ipsilateral fractures of the scapula and clavicle. J Trauma 1997;42(2):239–42.

[56] Hashiguchi H, Ito H. Clinical outcome of the treatment of floating shoulder by osteosynthesis for clavicular fracture alone. J Shoulder Elbow Surg 2003;12(6):589–91.

[57] Egol KA, Connor PM, Karunakar MA, et al. The floating shoulder: clinical and functional results. J Bone Joint Surg Am 2001;83-A(8):1188–94.

[58] Labler L, Platz A, Weishaupt D, et al. Clinical and functional results after floating shoulder injuries. J Trauma 2004;57(3):595–602.

[59] Oh W, Jeon IH, Kyung S, et al. The treatment of double disruption of the superior shoulder suspensory complex. Int Orthop 2002;26(3):145–9.

[60] Leung KS, Lam TP. Open reduction and internal fixation of ipsilateral fractures of the scapular neck and clavicle. J Bone Joint Surg Am 1993;75(7):1015–8.

[61] van Noort A, van der Werken C. The floating shoulder. Injury 2006;37(3):218–27.

[62] Obremskey WT, Lyman JR. A modified judet approach to the scapula. J Orthop Trauma 2004; 18(10):696–9.

[63] Oreck SL, Burgess A, Levine AM. Traumatic lateral displacement of the scapula: a radiographic sign of neurovascular disruption. J Bone Joint Surg Am 1984;66(5):758–63.

[64] Damschen DD, Cogbill TH, Siegel MJ. Scapulothoracic dissociation caused by blunt trauma. J Trauma 1997;42(3):537–40.

[65] Brucker PU, Gruen GS, Kaufmann RA. Scapulothoracic dissociation: evaluation and management. Injury 2005;36(10):1147–55.

[66] Ebraheim NA, Pearlstein SR, Savolaine ER, et al. Scapulothoracic dissociation (closed avulsion of the scapula, subclavian artery, and brachial plexus): a newly recognized variant, a new classification, and a review of the literature and treatment options. J Orthop Trauma 1987;1(1):18–23.

[67] Zelle BA, Pape HC, Gerich TG, et al. Functional outcome following scapulothoracic dissociation. J Bone Joint Surg Am 2004;86-A(1):2–8.

[68] Canadian Orthopedic Trauma Assocation. Nonoperative treatment compared with plate fixation of displaced midshaft clavicular fractures. A multicenter, randomized clinical trial. J Bone Joint Surg Am 2007;89(1):1–10.

[69] Goldstein LJ, Watson JM. Traumatic scapulothoracic dissociation: case report and literature review. J Trauma 2000;48(3):533–5.

[70] Sampson LN, Britton JC, Eldrup-Jorgensen J, et al. The neurovascular outcome of scapulothoracic dissociation. J Vasc Surg 1993;17(6):1083–8 [discussion: 1088–9].

ELSEVIER
SAUNDERS

Orthop Clin N Am 39 (2008) 475–482

ORTHOPEDIC
CLINICS
OF NORTH AMERICA

Management of Proximal Humeral Nonunions and Malunions

Emilie V. Cheung, MD[a], John W. Sperling, MD[b],*

[a]Department of Orthopedic Surgery, Stanford University, 300 Pasteur Dr,
Edwards R-155, Stanford, CA 94305-5335, USA
[b]Department of Orthopedic Surgery, Mayo Clinic, 200 First Street, SW, Rochester, MN 55905, USA

Proximal humeral fractures are one of the most common upper extremity fractures seen by orthopedic surgeons. In elderly patients, they are the third most common fracture after hip fractures and distal radius fractures [1]. The majority of proximal humerus fractures are nondisplaced or minimally displaced, and the functional outcome has been satisfactory in most [2]. In about 15% to 20% of these fractures, displacement is considered unacceptable, and surgery may be indicated to improve outcomes [2]. Treatment options for displaced fractures are controversial; there are many variations in clinical practice. A minority of these fractures treated with either open or closed treatment eventually develop into malunion or nonunion. Prevention of nonunion or malunion is possible by early recognition of fracture displacement with proper serial radiographs and close clinical follow-up, including serial true anterior-posterior views and axillary views of the shoulder. This review discusses the classification, treatment options, and reported outcomes of proximal humeral nonunions and malunions.

Proximal humeral nonunions

Nonunion of a fracture of the proximal humerus is uncommon, but it is often associated with severe shoulder dysfunction and pain. Proximal humeral nonunions may result from the initial displacement of the fracture, overly aggressive rehabilitation, and poor patient compliance. Patient comorbidities such as osteoporosis, alcoholism, tobacco use, mental illness, systemic use of corticosteroids, and rheumatoid arthritis may be associated with nonunion [3–5].

Interposition of soft tissue, such as the rotator cuff, biceps tendon, or deltoid muscle fibers, as well as synovial fluid at the fracture site may also lead to nonunion [6,7]. After operative treatment, a nonunion may develop if there has been inadequate fixation. Most often, nonunions of the proximal humerus involve two-part fractures at the surgical neck region [3,8]. Norris and colleagues [9] considered fractures of the proximal humerus that have not clinically healed in three months as nonunions.

Classification of nonunions of the proximal humerus

Because of differences in outcomes depending on the location of the nonunion site, Checchia and colleagues [6] proposed a classification system for nonunions of the proximal humerus. Nonunions of the surgical neck were divided into four groups. Group 1: High, 2-part nonunion, includes fractures of the anatomical neck with a very small proximal fragment. This includes cases of fractures in three parts in which the tuberosities are consolidated, with displacement of less than 5 mm. In such cases, internal fixation is very difficult to perform. Bone cavitation is seen at the proximal fragment because of rapid resorption of the cancellous bone under the humeral head. Neer [10] proposed that this rapid resorption occurs secondary to communication between the

* Corresponding author.
  E-mail address: sperling.john@mayo.edu
(J.W. Sperling).

fracture and the synovial fluid of the joint. Group 2: Low, 2-part nonunion, includes nonunions occurring between the lesser tuberosity and the insertion of the pectoralis major tendon with a larger proximal fragment than in group 1. This includes cases of fractures in three parts in which the tuberosities are consolidated, with displacement of less than 5 mm. The authors noted that the different bone quality in "high" versus "low" 2-part nonunions necessitates different surgical techniques. High nonunions often are associated with cavitation of the proximal fragment, which may preclude hardware placement and necessitate an arthroplasty procedure if surgical treatment is rendered. Group 3: Complex nonunion, includes nonunions secondary to three-part, four-part, or head-splitting fractures of the surgical neck and with displacement of the tuberosities greater than 5 mm. Group 4: Lost fragment nonunion, includes those after high-energy trauma, open fractures, or posttraumatic osteomyelitis of the proximal humerus.

Treatment

Nonoperative treatment may be appropriate for those patients who have minimal or no pain and satisfactory range of motion and function. A nonfunctional deltoid muscle is a relative contraindication for operative treatment because the reconstruction would be ultimately nonfunctional. Open reduction internal fixation is recommended for patients when the glenohumeral joint surface is maintained. Bone grafting may be used to augment fixation [8]. Arthroplasty is recommended when the articular surface is destroyed or when there is severe cavitation of the humeral head fragment precluding stable internal fixation [7].

Results of surgical treatment

Few reports in the literature discuss the results of surgical treatment for nonunions of the proximal humerus treated with different methods. Duralde and colleagues [7] reported satisfactory results in 55% of 20 nonunions treated with either open reduction internal fixation (ORIF) or hemiarthroplasty. There were 15 complications in the 20 patients, 11 of which needed reoperation. There was a relatively high reoperation rate in the ORIF group compared with the hemiarthroplasty group. Only half of the patients in the ORIF group obtained union at an average of 7 months. Nine of 10 patients in the ORIF group required reoperation because of hardware

removal, lysis of adhesions, or continued nonunion. Surgical reconstruction usually resulted in pain relief, but function and motion were fair to poor. Surgery should be considered carefully in terms of risks and benefits to the patient and should be reserved for those patients with significant disability.

Healy and colleagues [3] reported their results of 25 proximal humeral nonunions treated by four different methods. Overall results were fair, with less than half of the patients having good results. The worse results occurred with the use of flexible unreamed intramedullary nails; all five patients with this treatment had poor results. The best results were noted after open reduction internal fixation with a T-plate and tension band placed from the rotator cuff to the plate/humeral shaft composite with bone grafting. Proximal humeral arthroplasty was performed in six of the 25 patients, half of whom had a good result, and average forward elevation was only 72°. Similar to the prior study, pain relief was more consistently achieved, but function and motion were ultimately limited. Hemiarthroplasty was recommended in elderly patients whose poor bone quality precluded satisfactory bony purchase with internal fixation devices.

More recently, improved results with ORIF for proximal humeral nonunions have been reported. Ring and colleagues [11] reported healing in 92% of proximal humeral nonunions treated with a blade plate and autogenous bone grafting. Twenty of 25 patients reported good to excellent results. Twenty-three of the 25 patients had healing within 6 months. Good results of ORIF with bone grafting in a series of 13 patients was reported by Galatz and colleagues [8]. Blade plate fixation was used in ten patients, and T-plate fixation was used in three. Twelve of the 13 patients had an excellent or good result. Norris and colleagues [9] reported that range of motion improved more in those patients who underwent ORIF with intramedullary fixation and bone grafting for proximal humeral nonunions than those treated nonoperatively or those treated with hemiarthroplasty. Successful use of locking plate fixation with iliac crest bone grafting for proximal humeral nonunions has recently been reported (Figs. 1 and 2) [12].

The results of shoulder arthroplasty for a cohort of patients with proximal humeral nonunions at the Mayo Clinic were reported by Antuna and colleagues [13]. Twenty-one shoulders underwent hemiarthroplasty, and four

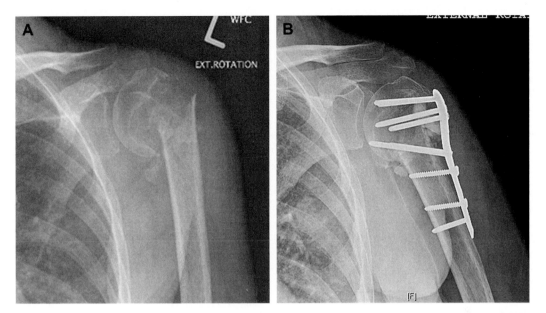

Fig. 1. (*A*) AP view of the shoulder shows a delayed union at the surgical neck in a 47-year-old woman 3.5 months after injury. (*B*) Postoperative radiograph at 3 months after osteosynthesis shows improved alignment and evidence of bone healing.

underwent total shoulder arthroplasty. Shoulder arthroplasty resulted in significant pain relief and improvement in motion, but results are inferior to those of arthroplasty for the primary indication of osteoarthritis. There were 12 excellent or satisfactory results and 13 unsatisfactory results. Similar to the prior studies, it was concluded

that function is not restored completely with arthroplasty, but pain relief and motion can be improved.

The reverse shoulder arthroplasty has been used successfully in treatment of failed hemiarthroplasty for proximal humeral fracture, tumor resection, rotator cuff tear arthropathy, and

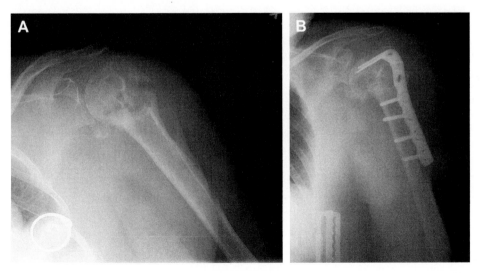

Fig. 2. (*A*) AP view of the shoulder in a 53-year-old woman with nonunion of proximal humeral fracture. (*B*) Postoperative radiograph after revision ORIF with blade plate fixation and autogenous and allogenic bone grafting.

fracture sequelae [14–18]. Its role in the treatment of proximal humeral nonunions has not yet been established clearly. The reverse shoulder prosthesis may be a reasonable treatment option in the elderly patient with a proximal humeral nonunion to alleviate pain relief and improve shoulder function as a salvage procedure (Fig. 3).

Proximal humeral malunions

One of the leading causes of poor shoulder function in patients with malunion of the proximal humerus is varus angulation of the humeral head in relation to the shaft. This may be related to the acceptance of unsuccessful closed reduction or imperfect open reduction internal fixation. Varus deformity of the proximal humerus causes limitations in active forward elevation and abduction caused by impingement of the greater tuberosity. The subacromial space is decreased in these shoulders, and the proximity of the greater tuberosity to the coracoacromial arch makes it prone to impingement. The sliding surface between the humeral head and the glenoid is also decreased. In addition, the proximity between the supraspinatus origin and insertion decreases

its lever arm, affecting shoulder function. Although some older patients are willing to accept functional limitations of shoulder elevation, many younger patients find this to be unacceptable.

Classification of proximal humeral malunion

A classification system for proximal humeral malunions proposed by Beredjiklian and colleagues [19] includes three types: type 1, malposition of the tuberosities; type 2, incongruity of articular surface; and type 3, articular fragment malposition. The authors emphasize that soft tissue pathology plays a major role in the functional impairment and stiffness seen in proximal humeral malunions. Both the bone and soft tissue pathology need to be corrected at the time of surgery to optimize outcome.

Arthroscopic treatment of proximal humeral malunion

Malposition of the tuberosities may be addressed arthroscopically. There has been one case report on the successful management of a medially displaced lesser tuberosity malunion that was causing a bony block to rotation with arthroscopic debridement and reshaping of the

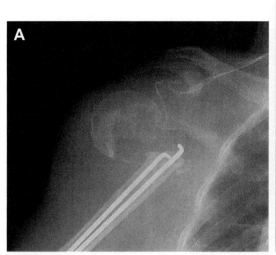
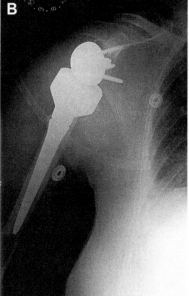

Fig. 3. (*A*) AP view of the shoulder in a 70-year-old woman with nonunion of the proximal humeral fracture at the surgical neck after attempted osteosynthesis. Note the cavitation in the proximal fragment. (*B*) Postoperative radiograph after reversed total shoulder arthroplasty. This patient had very minimal pain, active forward elevation of 90°, and external rotation of 30° 1 year postoperatively.

bone block. Arthroscopy is a useful tool for evaluation of the soft tissues and intra-articular abnormalities. In addition, capsular contractures or subacromial or subcoracoid impingement can be addressed. Two of the greater tuberosity malunions (type 1) reported by Beredjiklian and colleagues [19] were treated with arthroscopic acromioplasty. The authors note that the indication for acromioplasty is less than 15 mm displacement of the tuberosity. Burkhart [20] reported on arthroscopic subscapularis tenolysis for treating glenohumeral stiffness after ORIF of a displaced three-part proximal humerus fracture.

Corrective osteotomy of the proximal humerus

A limited number of reports in the literature discuss the surgical treatment of proximal humeral malunions. One of the therapeutic options is to correct the deformity with an osteotomy. This is indicated in younger, active patients who have no radiographic or clinical evidence of degenerative changes on the glenoid and humeral articular surfaces. In older, less active patients with evidence of degenerative joint disease, a joint replacement arthroplasty procedure may be more appropriate and definitive.

Indications for this procedure include patient dissatisfaction because of loss of active motion of the shoulder as well as impingement-type shoulder pain. Contraindications are massive irreparable rotator cuff tears; degenerative changes of the articular surfaces, including avascular necrosis; multiple angular deformities; active infection; or nerve injury.

Preoperative imaging studies, including true anterior-posterior (AP) and axillary radiographs of the shoulder are essential. It may be beneficial to obtain radiographs of the contralateral shoulder for comparison of the patient's neck-shaft angle. Computed tomography (CT) scans with three-dimensional (3-D) reconstructions may be useful in complex cases for preoperative planning.

Benegas and colleagues [21] described their preoperative planning and surgical technique of performing a laterally based closing wedge osteotomy for varus malunions of the proximal humerus. True AP views in external rotation of both shoulders are obtained. The neck-shaft angles are measured on the radiographs. The size of the bone wedge to be removed to obtain the patient's normal neck-shaft angle is calculated by comparison with the normal shoulder. The procedure is performed in the beachchair position

through a deltopectoral approach. The inferior aspect of the greater tuberosity is exposed. The closing wedge osteotomy is then performed, and internal fixation is achieved with a T plate. If there is an acromial process present, it may be beneficial to perform an acromioplasty to decrease the chance of postoperative impingement-type pain.

Results of correctional osteotomy of proximal humeral malunions have been reported by a few investigators. Benegas and colleagues [21] reported their results in five patients with varus malunions treated with valgus osteotomy of the surgical neck with osteosynthesis with plate and screws. The mean age of the patients was 53 years, and mean follow-up was 34 months. Four of the five patients had been treated initially nonoperatively. At 6 weeks after surgery, bony union was noted in all patients. All patients were satisfied with their result, and all but one was able to return to their previous occupation. All patients had significant improvements in forward elevation and pain relief. Complications included postoperative bleeding in one patient, which required a return to the operating room , and two patients eventually required hardware removal because of pain with shoulder flexion. There were no neurological complications.

Russo and colleagues [22] reported on 19 patients, mean age 46, who had posttraumatic malunion treated with three different types of osteotomies: osteotomy of the humeral neck for varus deformity, isolated osteotomy of the greater tuberosity, and a triplanar osteotomy for three- and four-fragment sequelae. Excellent results based on Constant scores were obtained in 14 and satisfactory results in five. All patients had improvement in range of motion and pain relief. Complications included one case of temporary axillary nerve neuropraxia and one case of complex regional pain syndrome, which resolved at 1 year. The authors caution that surgery is very technically challenging. Imperfect positioning of the greater or lesser tuberosities was noted in six cases, and resorption of the greater tuberosity and necrosis of the humeral head was noted in one case. The authors point out that their results were not inferior to those reported for hemiarthroplasty for proximal humeral malunions. This may be an effective treatment option for young, active patients in whom an arthroplasty would be contraindicated. If arthroplasty is needed in the future, good repositioning of the tuberosity may facilitate implantation of the prosthesis.

Arthroplasty for malunions of proximal humeral fractures

Arthroplasty for sequelae of proximal humeral fractures may be technically difficult. The shoulders tend to be stiff with distorted proximal humeral anatomy, soft tissue damage, subdeltoid adhesions, and rotator cuff tears. Avascular necrosis may be co-existent with malunion, and articular incongruence may be present.

A deltopectoral approach is used. The deltoid muscle and subscapularis may be atrophic in some cases. The subacromial, subdeltoid, and subcoracoid spaces are carefully freed of scar tissue. The joint capsule is released from the humerus as well as around the glenoid rim. The subscapularis is released from the scapular neck, and a Z-lengthening may be needed if external rotation is limited. Alternatively, a lesser tuberosity osteotomy with the subscapularis attached may be performed to improve mobilization. The rotator cuff integrity is assessed. Preparation of the humeral canal for placement of the prosthesis is performed. An osteotomy of the greater tuberosity is performed only if necessary for satisfactory placement of the prosthesis within the altered anatomy, but every effort is made to avoid performing the greater tuberosity osteotomy. Great care should be taken to leave enough bone attached to the rotator cuff to allow solid fixation of the tuberosities to the diaphysis. The rotator cuff is released on its articular and bursal surfaces to optimize excursion. After the

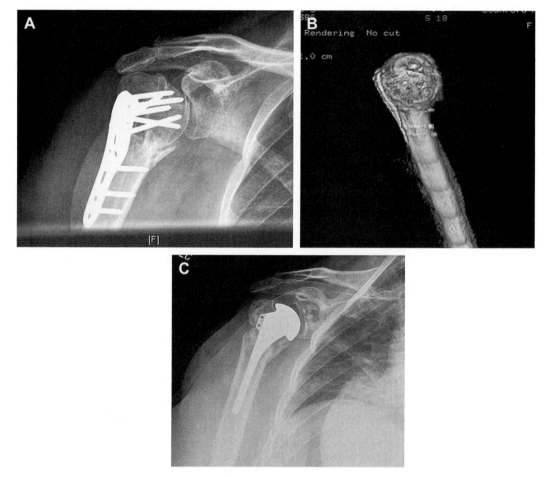

Fig. 4. (*A*) AP view of the shoulder in a 54-year-old woman with varus malunion at the surgical neck of the proximal humerus. (*B*) CT scan with 3-D reconstruction shows evidence of avascular necrosis of the humeral head with collapse of the articular surface. (*C*) Postoperative radiograph after total shoulder arthroplasty and acromioplasty. This patient had no pain, active forward elevation of 110°, and external rotation of 60° 1 year postoperatively.

prosthesis is placed, the tuberosities are fixed both to the implant and the humeral shaft with heavy nonabsorbable sutures. Autologous bone graft may be taken from the humeral head or iliac crest to augment fixation. Acromioplasty may be performed to improve the space under the coracoacromial arch.

The results in patients with old trauma are inferior to the results currently obtained in patients with primary osteoarthritis or those with four-part fractures treated in the acute setting. Pain relief is more reliably achieved postoperatively than motion. Mansat and colleagues [23] reported on 28 patients with sequelae of proximal humeral fractures treated with shoulder arthroplasty. Based on the Neer criteria, the results were satisfactory in only 64%. Mean active elevation was 107°, and 85% of patients reported no or slight pain. The final result was positively influenced by the integrity of the rotator cuff. Also, patients with acromiohumeral distances of greater than 8 mm had better results than those who did not. The authors conclude that the malunion of the greater tuberosity can be tolerated if it does not compromise acceptable positioning of the humeral component. However, if an osteotomy needs to be performed because of major displacement, results are unpredictable. All three patients who required a greater tuberosity osteotomy at the time of arthroplasty had an unsatisfactory result.

Similarly, Boileau [24] reported 42% good to excellent results in 71 patients who underwent shoulder arthroplasty for sequelae of proximal humeral fractures. They reported a 27% complication rate, including four diaphyseal fractures, one metaphyseal fracture, two cases of deep infection, one return to the operating room for acromioplasty, and one failure of fixation of the greater tuberosity. The most significant factor affecting results was the need for greater tuberosity osteotomy. All patients who underwent a greater tuberosity osteotomy were not able to regain active elevation above 90°. The authors emphasize that arthroplasty for the treatment of sequelae of proximal humeral fractures should be performed without a greater tuberosity osteotomy when possible. They believe that devascularization of the greater tuberosity, leading to tuberosity nonunion, migration, and resorption, is probably the reason for these poor results.

Antuna and colleagues [25] and Beredjiklian and colleagues [19] have reported similar results. Antuna and colleagues [25] reported that 10 of 24 of their patients who had greater tuberosity osteotomy had a complication related to tuberosity nonunion, malunion, or resorption. Implantation of the humeral component in slight varus or valgus was not associated with an increased incidence of humeral component loosening (Fig. 4). Humeral components with a modified curvature in the stem have been used with success in their experience. When the tuberosity is displaced 1.5 cm, it may be necessary to reposition it to avoid impingement.

Beredjiklian and colleagues [19] reported similar results, but emphasized that malunion of the proximal humerus often is accompanied by some soft tissue abnormality, such as soft tissue contracture, a tear of the rotator cuff, or subacromial impingement, in addition to distortion of the bony anatomy. Both osseous and soft tissue abnormalities need to be corrected at the time of surgery to improve the chances of a satisfactory result.

Summary

Surgical treatment of proximal humeral nonunions and malunions are technically challenging. Osteosynthesis with bone grafting for the treatment of nonunions is indicated in young, active patients with adequate bone stock in the proximal fragment and preservation of the glenohumeral articular surfaces. Corrective osteotomy may be a reasonable option for proximal humeral malunions in young patients without evidence of degenerative joint disease. Arthroplasty for proximal humerus nonunions and malunions has a guarded outcome because of limitations in shoulder motion, but pain relief is more consistently improved.

References

[1] Baron AA, Barrett JA, Karagas MR. The epidemiology of peripheral fractures. Bone 1996;18: 209S–13S.

[2] Neer CS. Displaced proximal humerus fractures: I. Classification and evaluation. J Bone Joint Surg Am 1970;52:1077–89.

[3] Healy WL, Jupiter JB, Kristiansen TK, et al. Nonunion of the proximal humerus. A review of 25 cases. J Orthop Trauma 1990;4:424–31.

[4] Smith AM, Sperling JW, Cofield RH. Complications of operative fixation of proximal humeral fractures in patients with rheumatoid arthritis American Shoulder and Elbow Surgeons. J Shoulder Elbow Surg 2005;14:559–64.

[5] Rose PS, Adams CR, Torchia ME, et al. Locking plate fixation for proximal humeral fractures: initial results with a new implant American Shoulder and Elbow Surgeons. J Shoulder Elbow Surg 2007;16: 202–7.

[6] Checchia SL, Doneux P, Miyazaki AN, et al. Classification of non-unions of the proximal humerus. Int Orthop 2000;24:217–20.

[7] Duralde XA, Flatow EL, Pollock RG, et al. Operative treatment of nonunions of the surgical neck of the humerus American Shoulder and Elbow Surgeons. J Shoulder Elbow Surg 1996;5:169–80.

[8] Galatz LM, Williams GR Jr, Fenlin JM Jr, et al. Outcome of open reduction and internal fixation of surgical neck nonunions of the humerus. Journal 2004;18:63–7.

[9] Norris TR, Turner JA, Bovil D. Nonunion of the upper humerus: an analysis of the etiology and treatment in 28 cases. In: Post M, Morrey BF, Hawkins RJ, editors. Surgery of the shoulder. Chicago, (IL): Mosby Year Book Inc; 1990. p. 63–7.

[10] Neer CS. Nonunion of the surgical neck of the humerus. Orthopaedic Transactions 1983;7:389.

[11] Ring D, McKee MD, Perey BH, et al. The use of a blade plate and autogenous cancellous bone graft in the treatment of ununited fractures of the proximal humerus. J Shoulder Elbow Surg 2001;10:501–7.

[12] Dwyer AJ, Patnaik S, Smibert JG. Nonunion of complex proximal humerus fractures treated with locking plate. Injury Extra 2007;38:409–13.

[13] Antuna SA, Sperling JW, Sanchez-Sotelo J, et al. Shoulder arthroplasty for proximal humeral nonunions American Shoulder and Elbow Surgeon. J Shoulder Elbow Surg 2002;11:114–21.

[14] Wall B, Walch G. Reverse shoulder arthroplasty for the treatment of proximal humeral fractures. Hand Clin 2007;23:425–30, v–vi.

[15] Wall B, Nove-Josserand L, O'Connor DP, et al. Reverse total shoulder arthroplasty: a review of results according to etiology. J Bone Joint Surg Am 2007;89:1476–85.

[16] Boileau P, Watkinson D, Hatzidakis AM, et al. Neer Award 2005: the grammont reverse shoulder prosthesis: results in cuff tear arthritis, fracture sequelae, and revision arthroplasty. J Shoulder Elbow Surg 2006;15:527–40.

[17] Frankle M, Levy JC, Pupello D, et al. The reverse shoulder prosthesis for glenohumeral arthritis associated with severe rotator cuff deficiency. A minimum two-year follow-up study of sixty patients surgical technique. J Bone Joint Surg Am 2006; 88(Suppl 1 Pt 2):178–90.

[18] Frankle M, Siegal S, Pupello D, et al. The reverse shoulder prosthesis for glenohumeral arthritis associated with severe rotator cuff deficiency. A minimum two-year follow-up study of sixty patients. J Bone Joint Surg Am 2005;87:1697–705.

[19] Beredjiklian PK, Iannotti JP, Norris TR, et al. Operative treatment of malunion of a fracture of the proximal aspect of the humerus. J Bone Joint Surg Am 1998;80:1484–97.

[20] Burkhart SS. Arthroscopic subscapularis tenolysis: a technique for treating refractory glenohumeral stiffness following open reduction and internal fixation of a displaced three-part proximal humerus fracture. Arthroscopy 1996;12:87–91.

[21] Benegas E, Zoppi Filho A, Ferreira Filho AA, et al. Surgical treatment of varus malunion of the proximal humerus with valgus osteotomy. J Shoulder Elbow Surg 2007;16:55–9.

[22] Russo R, Vernaglia Lombardi L, Giudice G, et al. Surgical treatment of sequelae of fractures of the proximal third of the humerus. The role of osteotomies. Chir Organi Mov 2005;90:159–69.

[23] Mansat P, Guity MR, Bellumore Y, et al. Shoulder arthroplasty for late sequelae of proximal humeral fractures. J Shoulder Elbow Surg 2004; 13:305–12.

[24] Boileau P, Trojani C, Walch G, et al. Shoulder arthroplasty for the treatment of the sequelae of fractures of the proximal humerus. J Shoulder Elbow Surg 2001;10:299–308.

[25] Antuna SA, Sperling JW, Sanchez-Sotelo J, et al. Shoulder arthroplasty for proximal humeral malunions: long-term results. J Shoulder Elbow Surg 2002;11:122–9.

ELSEVIER
SAUNDERS

Orthop Clin N Am 39 (2008) 483–490

ORTHOPEDIC
CLINICS
OF NORTH AMERICA

Neurovascular Injuries in Shoulder Trauma

Peter C. Zarkadas, MD, FRCS(C), Thomas W. Throckmorton, MD,
Scott P. Steinmann, MD*

Mayo Clinic, Department of Orthopaedic Surgery, 200 First Street SW, Rochester, MN 55905, USA

Although the incidence of neurovascular injury following shoulder trauma is relatively uncommon, a missed diagnosis may have serious clinical ramifications for the patient, and potential medicolegal implications for the treating surgeon. When treating these injuries with closed reduction or surgery the neural and vascular structures are at risk, and therefore a detailed and thorough baseline neurovascular status is essential before treatment. We suggest a systematic clinical approach when presented with trauma to the shoulder. This article provides an easily reproducible yet comprehensive approach to the diagnosis, identification, and treatment of neurovascular injuries following shoulder trauma.

Shoulder trauma can be classified based on the type of injury, which includes shoulder dislocation, proximal humeral fracture, traction injury to the brachial plexus, blunt soft tissue injury, and penetrating injury. Because of the proximity of the brachial plexus and axillary vessels to the proximal humerus these structures are particularly vulnerable following any shoulder trauma. The potential for injury to the brachial plexus, peripheral nerves, or the axillary artery or vein must be considered when initially evaluating and managing each case of shoulder trauma in the emergency.

Anatomy

A review of the anatomy of the brachial plexus and the relationship of the axillary artery and its branches to the proximal humerus is relevant to

this discussion. Any component of the brachial plexus is subject to injury following shoulder trauma. The peripheral nerves that may be injured include most commonly the axillary nerve and less commonly the musculocutaneous, suprascapular, long thoracic, and spinal accessory nerves. The roots and trunks of the brachial plexus are also subject to traction injury commonly seen following sporting injuries, or may be injured by penetrating trauma (Fig. 1).

The axillary nerve is the terminal branch of the posterior cord, and lies posterior to the axillary artery and anteroinferior to the subscapularis. It enters the quadrilateral space accompanied by the posterior humeral circumflex artery, which is bordered by the teres major and minor muscles, the proximal humerus, and the long head of the triceps. On exiting it splits into an anterior branch identified consistently 4 to 7 cm inferior to the anterolateral corner of the acromion and a posterior branch, which innervates the teres minor and posterior deltoid (Fig. 2).

The musculocutaneous nerve enters the coracobrachialis and biceps an average 5.6 cm and 10 cm below the coracoid, respectively. It courses between the biceps and brachialis sending off motor branches before terminating as the lateral antebrachial cutaneous nerve to the lateral forearm (Fig. 3).

The suprascapular nerve originates from the upper trunk and enters the supraspinatus fossa through the suprascapular notch under the superior transverse scapular ligament and gives motor branches to the supraspinatus muscle. On exiting the supraspinatus fossa through the spinoglenoid notch it gives off branches to innervate the posterior joint capsule and motor branches to the infraspinatus (Fig. 4).

_____

* Corresponding author.

   E-mail address: steinmann.scott@mayo.edu
(S.P. Steinmann).

doi:10.1016/j.ocl.2008.06.005

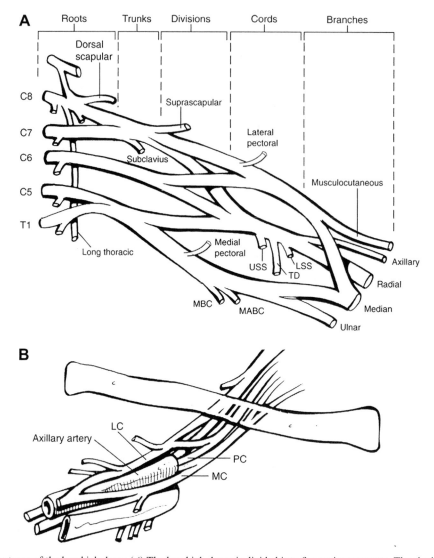

Fig. 1. Anatomy of the brachial plexus (*A*) The brachial plexus is divided into five major segments. The clavicle overlies the divisions. (*B*) The cords of the brachial plexus are named according to their anatomic relationship to the axillary artery. LC, lateral cord: LSS, lower subscapular nerve; MABC, medial antebrachiocutaneous nerve; MBC, medial brachiocutaneous nerve; MC, medial cord; PC, posterior cord; TD, thoracodorsal; USS, upper subscapular nerve. (*From:* Gill TJ, Hawkins RJ, editors. Complications of shoulder surgery: treatment and prevention. Philadelphia: Lippincott Williams and Wilkins; 2005. p. 91; with permission.)

The spinal accessory nerve (CN XI) supplies motor function to the trapezius and sternocleidomastoid muscles. It enters the neck through the jugular foramen, passing through the sternocleidomastoid, and innervates the underside of the trapezius. Most of the nerve function of the trapezius is derived from the spinal accessory nerve, although it does receive some innervation from cervical roots 3 and 4. The long thoracic nerve is a pure motor nerve derived from the cervical roots 5, 6, and 7 and is vulnerable to injury as it courses 26 cm along the lateral thorax innervating the serratus anterior.

The axillary artery is a continuation of the subclavian artery and is divided into three parts defined by the relationship to the pectoralis minor muscle. The anatomy of the axillary artery and its branches in relation to the proximal humerus puts it

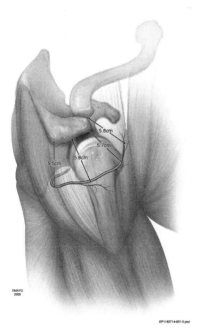

Fig. 2. Anatomy of the axillary nerve and its relationship to the acromion. The numbers refer to the average distance of the axillary nerve to the acromion. (*From:* Gill TJ, Hawkins RJ, editors. Complications of shoulder surgery: treatment and prevention. Philadelphia: Lippincott Williams and Wilkins; 2005. p. 86; with permission.)

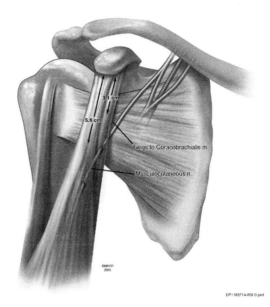

Fig. 4. Course of the suprascapular nerve through the suprascapular notch and the spinoglenoid notch. The distances represent the average distances of the nerve from the glenoid rim. (*From* Gill TJ, Hawkins RJ, editors. Complications of shoulder surgery: treatment and prevention. Philadelphia: Lippincott Williams and Wilkins; 2005. p. 87; with permission.)

at risk with any displaced fracture or dislocation. Injuries to the axillary artery most commonly occur at its third part where the subscapular and the anterior/posterior circumflex branch off.

Clinical evaluation

History

The mechanism of trauma should be carefully documented, whether low or high energy, blunt or penetrating; if possible the position of the arm at the time of injury should also be determined. Any pre-existing history of shoulder injury or dislocation should be explored with the patient. Hand dominance, occupation, and any previous surgery, especially involving the shoulder, should be carefully documented. The patient should be questioned about numbness or weakness of the involved extremity and the specific location, onset, and character of the pain.

It is not uncommon during patient evaluation in the emergency situation that a comprehensive history and physical examination is not possible because of the patient's state of confusion, sedation, or lack of consciousness. In this instance

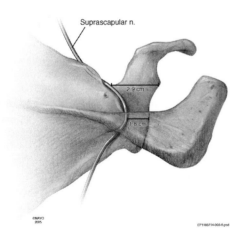

Fig. 3. Course of the musculocutaneous nerve and its relationship to the coracoid. The distances on the figure represent the highest branch entry point (3.1 cm) and the average entry point of the musculocutaneous nerve proper as it enters of the coracobrachialis (5.6 cm). (*From:* Gill TJ, Hawkins RJ, editors. Complications of shoulder surgery: treatment and prevention. Philadelphia: Lippincott Williams and Wilkins; 2005. p. 86; with permission.)

collateral information becomes important, as does a delayed comprehensive physical examination.

Physical examination

The first step in any trauma situation is to follow the advanced trauma life support protocol and stabilize the patient from an airway, breathing, and circulatory status before commencing an assessment of the involved extremity. If the injury involves or is suspected to involve the upper extremity and specifically the shoulder joint the first step is to properly expose the entire extremity, including exposing the cervical spine and the scapula during the log roll and examining and palpating for tenderness in that area.

It is recommended to organize the physical examination of the involved shoulder in a systematic and reproducible manner so that an occult neurovascular injury is not missed. The priority from a trauma standpoint is to assess the vascular supply of the upper extremity, which involves simply noting the color of the skin and palpating for a radial pulse, and noting its character and strength. If the pulse is weak or absent, capillary refill can be assessed, and a portable ultrasound of the radial, ulnar, and brachial arteries should be performed. The presence of a strong distal pulse does not exclude a vascular injury because the collateral network of vessels in the upper extremity may preserve distal blood flow. Physical signs that may also indicate an underlying vascular injury include an axillary hematoma, an expanding mass, bruits, and excessive bruising over the lateral chest wall. Paresthesia in the entire hand is often the most reported sign of inadequate perfusion to the extremity. A brachial:brachial index may also be performed to assist in the evaluation.

A detailed and systematic upper extremity neurologic examination should also be performed. If the patient presents with neck pain or is known to have prior cervical pathology careful attention must be paid to distinguish peripheral nerve involvement versus objective physical findings in a dermatomal or myotomal distribution. It is imperative to carefully document each peripheral nerve function for motor and sensory distribution. This documentation specifically includes the median, ulnar, radial, musculocutaneous, and axillary nerves. The examination can begin distally and progress proximally assessing for light touch and pinprick, and motor function at the hand, elbow, and shoulder compared with the contralateral side. Loss of any one of these nerves distally may guide the proximal examination. For example, loss of radial nerve function should make the examiner look closely at the axillary function because both are derived from the posterior cord.

Deltoid function is of particular significance to the shoulder in the trauma situation. Even in the case of a painful proximal humeral fracture or dislocation, the patient is asked to abduct, flex, and extend the arm against resistance while palpating the deltoid for contraction. The examination may be clouded by the patient's pain, but an attempt must be made and careful observation is needed to detect muscle firing. What can be assessed more consistently in a coherent patient is the sensory examination of the axillary nerve for light touch and pinprick in its autogenous area over the deltoid. Occasionally, sensation is preserved while the motor branch is compromised and therefore axillary nerve injury cannot be ruled out on the basis of normal sensation. If the axillary nerve cannot be properly assessed then this should be recorded in the medical record, and later reassessed. After any reduction maneuver for a shoulder fracture or dislocation, the upper extremity examination should be repeated and documented because reduction maneuvers have been implicated in nerve and vascular injuries [1–3].

Depending on the clinical scenario, and relevant to some shoulder injuries, are injuries of the suprascapular nerve, the spinal accessory nerve, and the long thoracic nerve. These injuries often present delayed, as they are not routinely examined in the emergency setting. The suprascapular nerve, which innervates the supraspinatus and infraspinatus, is examined by asking a patient to abduct then externally rotate their shoulder against resistance. The spinal accessory nerve innervates the trapezius, which can be examined by asking the patient to shrug the shoulder upward against resistance comparing strength side to side. The long thoracic nerve, which innervates the serratus anterior, often manifests in winging of the scapula and can be examined by forward flexing the arm, such as in a wall push-up.

Classification of nerve injury

Neurovascular injuries can be classified either based on anatomic location or on degree of nerve injury. Anatomically lesions can be described as supraclavicular or infraclavicular. Supraclavicular lesions generally involve avulsion of the nerve roots, carry a poor prognosis, and are generally not amenable to surgical treatment. Infraclavicular lesions have a more favorable prognosis and may be amenable to neurolysis or nerve grafting if recovery does not occur [4].

Nerve injuries have been described historically using the Seddon and Sunderland classification, which describes three possibilities for a nerve injury: neurapraxia, axonotmesis, or neurotmesis [5]. A neurapraxia is believed to be present when there is a conduction block at the site of nerve injury but no obvious visual injury to the nerve. The recovery time from the neurapraxia may be only hours if there is a traction neuropathy or potentially a few months depending on the severity of the injury to the myelin covering.

In axonotmesis, the nerve fibers have physically been disrupted; however, the epineurium and the perineurium remain intact preserving a conduit for nerve regeneration. Nerve recovery typically occurs at a rate of 1 to 4 mm per day. In neurotmesis, the nerve itself is physically disrupted and because of this, axonal continuity is severely disrupted. In such a nerve injury surgical intervention is required to obtain any meaningful functional outcome.

Neurologic injury

Axillary nerve

The axillary nerve is the most commonly injured nerve following shoulder trauma and is often associated with a combined brachial plexus injury. Paralysis of the axillary nerve is the most common complication of shoulder dislocation, occurring in 5% to 10% of these injuries. Additionally, as many as 54% of shoulder dislocations may have a subclinical axillary nerve lesion detectable by electromyography/nerve conduction studies (EMG/NCS) [6]. Fortunately, most axillary nerve lesions recover during their rehabilitation phase and are not clinically significant. Patients who are at higher risk for permanent injury include those older than the age of 50 and patients whose dislocation remains unreduced for more than 12 hours.

Blunt trauma is also known to cause injury to the axillary nerve by direct compression on the deep surface of the deltoid reported following a football and hockey injury [7]. In this study, nerve exploration in the setting of blunt trauma did not improve outcome and therefore is not indicated [8]. Penetrating trauma, on the other hand, with an associated axillary nerve involvement should be explored early.

An initial conservative approach is indicated in most axillary nerve injuries for the first 3 months following shoulder trauma. At 3 to 4 weeks a baseline EMG/NCS may be obtained. In a study of 77 patients following shoulder trauma, 33% of whom had axillary nerve involvement (9 complete and 15 partial), all had full recovery of function [9]. The initial conservative approach to treatment is advocated because most patients do well with nonoperative treatment. If the patient has no clinical or EMG improvement by 6 to 9 months then patients should be referred for surgical exploration with neurolysis and possibly nerve grafting. If patients who have axillary nerve paralysis present late (more than 12 months) the result of nerve graft and nerve repair is poor.

Musculocutaneous nerve

Musculocutaneous nerve injury is often associated with severe brachial plexus palsy and rarely presents in isolation. Isolated injuries may occur from a penetrating injury or blunt trauma to the coracoid. Musculocutaneous nerve traction injury may be seen following glenohumeral dislocation, but rarely in open injuries. Most palsies present as a mixed motor and sensory deficit with weakness of elbow flexion and pain and numbness along the lateral forearm. Occasionally a pure sensory syndrome exists, which is exacerbated by elbow extension as the nerve is compressed between the biceps and brachialis. If a musculocutaneous injury is identified, observation and serial reassessment starting at 3 to 4 weeks with an EMG/NCS is used to establish a baseline. If there is no recovery of elbow flexion at 6 to 9 months then surgical exploration and neurolysis with nerve graft interposition should be attempted. When patients present late (more than 1 year following trauma) without nerve recovery, they may be candidates for a tendon transfer.

Suprascapular nerve

The suprascapular nerve is indispensable for proper shoulder function and a deficit may lead to loss of shoulder abduction and external rotation. It may mimic an acute rotator cuff tear and should be differentiated by EMG/NCS and an MRI of the shoulder. Suprascapular nerve injury can be the result of blunt trauma or fracture of the scapula. The injury may be a result of a traction injury as a twisting motion to the shoulder.

Patients may complain of pain of the posterior aspect of the shoulder and weakness in abduction and external rotation. Arthroscopic or open surgical exploration and decompression may be warranted if the suprascapular nerve is deemed compressed by scar or fracture. Late treatment with a latissimus tendon transfer may also be warranted.

Spinal accessory nerve

A spinal accessory nerve injury can result from blunt or penetrating trauma to the posterior shoulder or neck region. The resultant trapezius palsy can be debilitating to patients, because the trapezius is the predominant stabilizer of the scapula. Loss of function of the trapezius causes the shoulder to droop, allowing the scapula to rotate downward, outward, and away from the midline resulting in lateral winging. This winging can cause subacromial impingement and rotator cuff tendinopathy. Lateral winging of the scapula can also cause pain, decreased shoulder range of motion, and significantly altered physical appearance.

This condition is best diagnosed by initial EMG/NCS done at 3 to 4 weeks postinjury and every 2 to 3 months until clinical resolution or improvement in EMG/NCS results. Surgical exploration and neurotization may be performed after 6 months. When patients present late (more than 12 months) repair of the nerve is generally not useful, and an Eden-Lange trapezius reconstruction procedure may be considered. This operation involves a transfer of the levator scapulae to the scapular spine, rhomboid major onto the infraspinatus fossa, and the rhomboid minor to the supraspinatus fossa, with good cosmetic and functional results [10].

Long thoracic nerve

The long thoracic nerve is a pure motor nerve innervating the serratus anterior that plays an important role in stabilizing the scapula and preventing medial winging. The winging is different than that caused by spinal accessory nerve palsy, in that the scapula translates medially, with rotation of the inferior angle to the midline. The deformity becomes accentuated by forward flexion of the shoulder and is associated with pain and weakness. The best test for a long thoracic nerve palsy is EMG/NCS; treatment of a serratus nerve palsy is generally conservative and most generally resolve. After 12 months, if the patient is

severely affected by persistent scapular winging, a muscle transfer procedure may be considered. In this procedure the sternal head of the pectoralis muscle is transferred to the inferior scapular border and the reconstruction is augmented with tendon grafting with reasonable results [11,12]. Scapulothoracic fusion is also an option as a salvage procedure for both types of winging caused by a long thoracic nerve injury or a spinal accessory nerve injury.

Athletic injuries

Traction injuries to the brachial plexus are commonly seen following sporting injuries and have been the subject of several recent reviews [4,8,13,14]; these injuries are not described in this article. Suffice it say that that several conditions have been described among athletes, which include cervical radiculitis, brachial neuritis, and the burner (stinger).

Electrodiagnostic studies

Electrodiagnostic studies are helpful for diagnosis and preoperative planning. They can help confirm the diagnosis, give information on the location of the injury, and define the type of axonal loss that may exist, and can be used to decide whether to proceed with operative intervention.

Baseline EMG/NCS is best performed within 3 to 4 weeks after injury to a shoulder nerve. Follow-up serial electrodiagnostic studies performed with a repeat physical examination every 2 to 3 months helps document potential ongoing reinnervation. Denervation patterns seen on electromyography can be seen as early as 10 to 14 days after injury in proximally innervated muscles and 3 to 6 months postinjury in more distal muscles. A loss of motor unit potential recruitment can be demonstrated immediately after weakness is noted from a lower motor neuron injury. The detection of active motor units with voluntary effort and occasional fibrillations at rest is a good prognostic indicator compared with an absence of motor units and many fibrillations.

Typically, nerve conduction studies are also performed at the time of EMG. EMG studies can show evidence of early recovery in muscles. These electrical findings may occur before clinically apparent recovery begins to be noticed. An improvement in the EMG study does not necessarily equal a clinical recovery. Rather, a positive improvement in the electromyographic study indicates that an unknown number of nerve fibers have reached the muscle target and re-established a motor endplate connection.

Vascular injury

Arterial injuries around the shoulder are potentially limb- and even sometimes life-threatening [15–17], and every effort should be made to restore vascularity promptly to the upper limb. A well-perfused limb does not necessarily preclude a vascular injury, because an extensive network of collateral vessels may preserve distal pulses. A high level of awareness should therefore be maintained following every shoulder dislocation or displaced proximal humeral fracture. The artery can be injured by complete transection, intimal tear, avulsion of one or more branches, or an intravascular thrombus in these injuries. In addition to the arterial injury, venous injury can also occur whereby patients may present with a painful arm and unilateral swelling. Venography is indicated in this instance.

In the setting of an ischemic limb, an attempt should be made in the emergency room to reduce the dislocation or grossly displaced fracture under conscious sedation. If there is concern for an arterial injury, an angiogram of the involved extremity should be arranged and a vascular surgeon consulted. Patients who have objective evidence for an arterial injury either clinically or from an angiogram should be taken to the operating room for fracture fixation followed by vascular repair. An angiogram is an essential component of the work-up not only to confirm the diagnosis but also to localize the lesion and the extent of damage to the artery.

The timing of surgical intervention is determined largely by the ischemia time. The vascular occlusion itself may cause permanent neurologic deficits and therefore timely vascular surgical repair is necessary. It is necessary to stabilize the fracture first with internal fixation following reduction because motion and manipulation may endanger the vascular repair. If limb ischemia time has been greater than 6 hours, a prophylactic forearm fasciotomy should be performed, which would include a release from the antecubital fossa to the carpal tunnel. Postoperatively patients should be carefully monitored and regular checks of the neurovascular status of the affected limb performed. If limb ischemia has been prolonged without prophylactic fasciotomy the patient should be carefully monitored for a compartment syndrome of the forearm.

Vascular injury following fracture

The incidence of vascular injury following four-part proximal humeral fractures was reported in one series of 81 patients to be 4.9% [18]. Vascular injuries are rarely seen in minimally displaced fractures, however [19]. Vascular injuries following proximal humeral fracture can also present delayed as a pseudoaneurysm and mass in the shoulder region [20].

Vascular injury following dislocation

The mechanism by which the axillary artery is damaged by dislocation relates to the relative tautness of the artery as it exits under the pectoralis minor, especially in abduction and external rotation. When the shoulder dislocates anteriorly it pushes the artery forward, increasing the tension with potential subsequent rupture. The third part of the axillary artery is most frequently injured just proximal to the division of the anterior circumflex artery [21]. The risk factors that predispose to an axillary arterial injury include a history of recurrent dislocation (27% of cases) and older age (86% of patients older than 50) [22]. The reported incidence of vascular injury following shoulder dislocation in a multicenter retrospective analysis was 0.97% [23].

Injury to the artery may occur at the time of dislocation or even from the relocation maneuver [1–3]. It must be stressed that a reduction in an elderly patient who has a chronic dislocation is potentially dangerous. Calvert and colleagues [15] in 1941 reported a mortality of 50% in 64 of 91 cases of reduction performed many weeks after initial dislocation. A vascular injury should be suspected in any case of posterior sternoclavicular dislocation or in the rare case of scapulothoracic dissociation [24,25].

Summary

Although the incidence of neurovascular injuries is uncommon the ramifications of a missed injury are potentially devastating to the patient. A thorough physical examination and low threshold for investigation if there is any concern of a neurovascular injury can protect the patient and treating surgeon.

References

[1] Curr JF. Rupture of the axillary artery complicating dislocation of the shoulder. Report of a case. J Bone Joint Surg Br 1970;52(2):313–7.

[2] Antal CS, Conforty B, Engelberg M, et al. Injuries to the axillary due to anterior dislocation of the shoulder. J Trauma 1973;13(6):564–6.

[3] Gugenheim S, Sanders RJ. Axillary artery rupture caused by shoulder dislocation. Surgery 1984;95(1): 55–8.

[4] Silliman JF, Dean MT. Neurovascular injuries to the shoulder complex. J Orthop Sports Phys Ther 1993; 18(2):442–8.

[5] Seddon H. Three types of nerve injury. Brain 1943; 66:238–88.

[6] Travlos J, Goldberg I, Boome RS. Brachial plexus lesions associated with dislocated shoulders. J Bone Joint Surg Br 1990;72(1):68–71.

[7] Perlmutter GS, Leffert RD, Zarins B. Direct injury to the axillary nerve in athletes playing contact sports. Am J Sports Med 1997;25(1):65–8.

[8] Koffler KM, Kelly JDt. Neurovascular trauma in athletes. [erratum appears in Orthop Clin North Am. 2003 Jan;34(1):xiii]. Orthop Clin North Am 2002;33(3):523–34.

[9] Blom S, Dahlback LO. Nerve injuries in dislocations of the shoulder joint and fractures of the neck of the humerus. A clinical and electromyographical study. Acta Chir Scand 1970;136(6):461–6.

[10] Wiater JM, Bigliani LU. Spinal accessory nerve injury. Clin Orthop Relat Res 1999;368:5–16.

[11] Wiater JM, Flatow EL. Long thoracic nerve injury. Clin Orthop Relat Res 1999;368:17–27.

[12] Steinmann SP, Wood MB. Pectoralis major transfer for serratus anterior paralysis. J Shoulder Elbow Surg 2003;12(6):555–60.

[13] Aval SM, Durand P Jr, Shankwiler JA. Neurovascular injuries to the athlete's shoulder: part I. J Am Acad Orthop Surg 2007;15(4):249–56.

[14] Aval SM, Durand P Jr, Shankwiler JA. Neurovascular injuries to the athlete's shoulder: part II. J Am Acad Orthop Surg 2007;15(5):281–9.

[15] Calvert J, Lmal L. Luxations de l'epaule et lesions vasculaires. J Chir 1942;58:337–46 [in French].

[16] Zuckerman JD, Flugstad DL, Teitz CC, et al. Axillary artery injury as a complication of proximal humeral fractures. Two case reports and a review of the literature. Clin Orthop Relat Res 1984;189: 234–7.

[17] Lodding P, Angeras U. Fatal axillary artery injury following anterior dislocation of the shoulder. Ann Chir Gynaecol 1988;77(3):125–7.

[18] Stableforth PG. Four-part fractures of the neck of the humerus. J Bone Joint Surg Br 1984;66(1): 104–8.

[19] Hayes JM, Van Winkle GN. Axillary artery injury with minimally displaced fracture of the neck of the humerus. J Trauma 1983;23(5):431–3.

[20] Harris O, Roche CJ, Torregliani WC, et al. Delayed presentation of pseudoaneurysm complicating closed humeral fracture: MR diagnosis. Skeletal Radiol 2001;30(11):648–51.

[21] Onyeka W. Anterior shoulder dislocation: an unusual complication. Emerg Med J 2002;19(4): 367–8.

[22] Gates JD, Knox JB. Axillary artery injuries secondary to anterior dislocation of the shoulder. J Trauma 1995;39(3):581–3.

[23] Sparks SR, DeLaRosa J, Bergan JJ, et al. Arterial injury in uncomplicated upper extremity dislocations. Ann Vasc Surg 2000;14(2):110–3.

[24] Katsamouris AN, Kafetzakis A, Kostas T, et al. The initial management of scapulothoracic dissociation: a challenging task for the vascular surgeon. Eur J Vasc Endovasc Surg 2002;24(6):547–9.

[25] Syed AA, Williams HR. Shoulder disarticulation: a sequel of vascular injury secondary to a proximal humeral fracture. Injury 2002;33(9):771–4.

Orthop Clin N Am 39 (2008) 491–505

Management of Acute Clavicle Fractures

Won Kim, MD, Michael D. McKee, MD, FRCS(C)*

*Division of Orthopaedic Surgery, St. Michaels Hospital and the University of Toronto,
55 Queen Street East, Suite 800, Ontario M5C 1R6, Canada*

It has been believed since the time of Hippocrates that clavicle fractures require little more than benign neglect by clinicians [1]. Although many patients who have clavicle injuries do achieve adequate healing and functional recovery without surgical interventions, good outcomes, especially with displaced fractures, are not universal. Recent literature suggests that a subset of midclavicular injuries may warrant primary surgical treatment to minimize the incidence of non-union and/or symptomatic malunion. Furthermore, certain types of clavicular injuries have been shown to result in suboptimal outcomes when managed nonoperatively. This article is based on the currently available clinical evidence on the evolving management of acute clavicle fractures.

Epidemiology

Clavicle fractures are one of the most common fractures encountered in orthopedic practice. Previous epidemiologic studies suggest that clavicle fractures represent up to 5% of all adult fractures and up to 44% of all shoulder girdle fractures [2–4]. The overall incidence of the injury was estimated to be 29 to 64 per 100 000 population per year in two large European series [5,6]. The incidence of the injury also is characterized by a bimodal age distribution with peaks under age 40 years and above age 70 years. The typical young male patient sustains a high-energy clavicle fracture secondary to a fall from height, a direct blow during a sporting event, or a motor vehicle

collision (Fig. 1) [4–6]. The increased incidence in the elderly is found in both men and women and represents low-energy or insufficiency fractures caused by a fall from a standing height [3,6]. Contemporary series also report a relatively high proportion of clavicle injuries as a result of high-energy trauma or polytrauma from sports, falls, and motor vehicle collisions (Fig. 2) [4–9]. This trend probably reflects the changing demographics of the modern society with greater participation in sports and high-risk behaviors than seen many decades ago.

With respect to the incidence of different fracture types, fractures of the middle third of the clavicle are by far the most common, accounting for 69% to 81% of all clavicle fractures [2–8]. Of these, 48% to 73% are displaced fractures. The second most common type is fracture of the lateral or distal third of the clavicle, accounting for 16% to 30% of all clavicle fractures [2–8]. Of these, 10% to 52% are displaced. Less than 3% of all clavicle fractures are fractures of the medial or proximal third of the clavicle [2–8].

Applied anatomy

In human embryology, the clavicle is the first bone to ossify; its ossification begins during the fifth week of gestation [10]. It also contains the last ossification center to fuse in human body: the medial ossification center adjacent to the sternoclavicular (SC) joint fuses well past 20 years of age [10,11]. This late fusion of the medial physis explains the pathophysiology behind the physeal separation injuries seen in young adults.

Morphologically, the clavicle is a subcutaneous, S-shaped long bone with an anterior apex medially and posterior apex laterally [10,12]. It

* Corresponding author.
E-mail address: mckeem@smh.toronto.on.ca
(M.D. McKee).

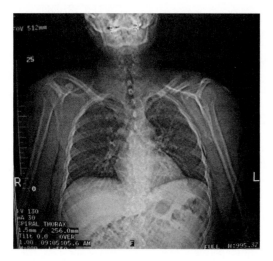

Fig. 1. A CT scan scout view demonstrates severe displacement of a mid-shaft fracture of the clavicle following high-speed vehicular trauma. Such displacement in a young, active individual is a relative indication for primary operative fixation.

widens at both the sternal and the acromion ends, transitioning through the narrower tubular middle third. The medial third of the clavicle has a relatively flat superior border. It articulates with the sternum through the strong capsuloligamentous attachments at the SC joint and the first rib. Attached to the medial third of the clavicle are the sternocleidomastoid, the pectoralis major, and the sternohyoid muscles. The sternocleidomastoid muscle provides the major deforming force on the medial fragment, pulling superomedially in a midshaft fracture of the clavicle [13,14]. The wide lateral third of the clavicle contains the apex of the superior bow of the clavicle. It is anchored solidly to the scapula by the

acromioclavicular (AC) capsulo-ligament and the coracoclavicular (CC) ligaments—the trapezoid ligament laterally and the conoid ligament medially. Attached to the lateral third of the clavicle are the anterior fibers of the deltoid and the trapezius muscles in addition to the clavicular head of the pectoralis major muscle. The pectoralis major and the weight of the arm provide the major deforming force on the lateral fragment, pulling inferomedially and anteriorly in fractures of the middle third of the clavicle [13,14]. A thorough understanding of the osseous morphology and of the deforming forces applied to different clavicle-fracture fragments is essential for determining the appropriate therapeutic intervention and mode of fixation, as discussed later in the section on management.

Overlying the clavicle and its attached muscles are the branches of supraclavicular nerves and the platysma muscle. During a surgical exposure of the clavicle, the platysma must be divided. Just deep to it are the supraclavicular nerves branches over the medial and middle thirds of the clavicle [13,15]. The authors advocate identifying and protecting these cutaneous nerves during the surgical exposure to prevent dysesthesia after the surgery [15].

Functionally, the clavicle acts as a strut that connects the shoulder girdle to the axial skeleton. Clinical and biomechanical studies demonstrate the importance of restoring and maintaining the normal length of this strut, and hence the attached muscle unit length, to optimize the functional recovery of the shoulder girdle following a clavicle fracture [14,16–20]. The clavicle also protects the vital neurovascular bundles coursing underneath it as well as the apex of the lung. The brachial plexus and the subclavian vessels traverse toward the axillae under the middle third of the clavicle,

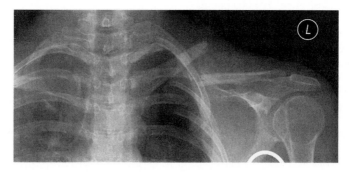

Fig. 2. Multiple rib fractures with associated pneumothorax in a patient who has a displaced mid-shaft clavicle fracture. Associated injuries are common with severely displaced clavicle fractures.

which forms the inferior border of the posterior triangle of the neck [13]. Medially, the carotid and jugular vessels are protected adjacent to the SC joint. Because of this intimate anatomic relationship between the clavicle and the neurovascular structures, a number of cases have been reported involving neurovascular compromise secondary to clavicle fractures [21–25].

The motion of the clavicle is interconnected intimately with the motion of the shoulder girdle through its articulation with the scapula. The SC joint serves as a stable medial pivot point on which the clavicle elevates and rotates, depending on the motion of the arm at the shoulder joint. Previous studies showed that, with the shoulder abduction and forward flexion, the clavicle can elevate as much as 15° to 30° and can rotate posteriorly 30° to 50° [26–29]. This close dynamic relationship between the clavicle and shoulder motion is well supported by clinical studies showing deficits in shoulder function after a clavicle malunion with shortening [14,20,26,28].

Mechanism of injury

Most clavicle fractures result from a fall or from a direct blow to the shoulder. This compressive force onto the clavicle is estimated to account for more than 85% of all clavicle fractures [5–8,29]. The middle third of the clavicle is the thinnest segment of the bone and is devoid of any protective muscular or ligamentous attachment, rendering it the weakest point of the bone; therefore clavicle fractures most commonly involve the middle third of the clavicle [2–8,29]. No studies to date have proposed any definite correlation between the mechanism of injury and the fracture location on the clavicle.

Much less common are fractures resulting from blunt or penetrating injuries directly to the clavicle. They can result from direct blows to the clavicle during sports activities, from seat belt injuries, or from ballistic injuries and are estimated to account for approximately 10% of clavicle fractures [5–8,29]. An even rarer mechanism of injury is a severe distraction injury around the shoulder girdle as seen in a scapulothoracic dissociation with distraction of the clavicle fracture site [30]. Because of the clavicle's close proximity to the neck and the chest, pathologic clavicle fractures from metastatic lung, breast, and neck cancers or previous irradiation and from primary neoplasms also have been reported without any

history of trauma [31–33]. In addition, stress fractures involving the clavicle have been reported [34,35].

Classification

A number of classification systems have been devised based on the location and the complexity of the fractures involving the clavicle. These classification systems aim to facilitate description of the fracture patterns and communication among surgeons in both clinical and research settings [6,36–39].

The first widely used classification system for clavicle fractures was introduced by Allman in 1967 [36]. This scheme divided the clavicle into three equal segments: group I (fractures of the middle third of the clavicle), group II (fractures of the lateral third of the clavicle), and group III (fractures of the medial third of the clavicle). This classification is simple to use and is designated in the order of decreasing frequency of fractures but does not address fracture pattern.

In 1968, Neer [37] added three subtypes to address the fractures of the lateral third of the clavicle that seemed to behave quite differently from those involving more medial segments. Recognizing the importance of an intact CC ligament in maintaining fracture stability, he divided fractures of the lateral third of the clavicle into three subtypes: type I (intact CC ligament), type II (CC ligament torn off the medial fragment), and type III (intra-articular fractures involving the AC joint with intact CC ligament). Rockwood [38] later emphasized the significance of an intact conoid ligament by subdividing Neer type II injuries.

Craig [39] then merged and modified the Allman and Neer classification systems by further subdividing fractures of the medial and lateral thirds of the clavicle and including periosteal and epiphyseal injuries. The Craig classification describes five subtypes of fractures of the medial and lateral thirds of the clavicle: type I (undisplaced), type II (displaced), type III (intra-articular), type IV (epiphyseal separation), and type V (comminuted). Nordqvist and Petersson [5] further classified the most frequent fractures of the middle third of the clavicle (Allman group I) as undisplaced, displaced, or comminuted fractures.

The most recent classification scheme proposed by Robinson [6] in 1998 is based on 1000 consecutive clavicle fractures seen over 6 years in

Edinburgh, Scotland. In his series, Robinson redesignated the fracture types from the medial to lateral direction: type I (fractures of the medial third of the clavicle), type II (fractures of the middle third of the clavicle), and type III (fractures of the lateral third of the clavicle). Fracture patterns such as displacement, angulation, comminution and extension into the SC or AC joint were considered in the subgrouping of each type. Although complicated, this classification system revealed prognostic value based on the initial fracture patterns, and both inter- and intraobserver reliability were high among orthopedic trainees. The main limitation of these classification systems is their lack of clear prognostic and therapeutic value. Further studies are warranted to improve these deficiencies.

Clinical evaluation

Most patients have a history of a direct fall onto the shoulder [4–6,8,29]. Because of its subcutaneous nature, the initial diagnosis of a clavicle fracture usually is readily apparent. In the context of a high-energy trauma or in a multiply injured patient, however, identifying associated injuries is much more challenging and is of great importance. Multiple studies have shown associated rib, scapular, intrathoracic, and neurovascular injuries, particularly to subclavian vessels and brachial plexus, in high-energy clavicle fractures [3,9,21–25].

On physical examination, inspection of the injured clavicle often reveals a tender, bony protuberance under the skin, ecchymosis, and swelling at the fracture site. Prolonged skin tenting may lead to skin necrosis and a secondarily open fracture. The ipsilateral shoulder may demonstrate a typical droop or ptosis with associated scapular anterior rotation or winging and a shortened clavicle [14,20,26]. A sizable and/or expanding hematoma around the fracture site may indicate an injury to the subclavian vessels that necessitates an inspection for a local bruit, diminished or absent distal pulses, and asymmetrical blood pressure measurements in the arms. A thorough neurologic examination is mandatory.

Radiologic evaluation

For an isolated clavicle injury, routine radiograph starts with a full-length antero-posterior view of the clavicle, which includes the SC and AC joints as well as the shoulder girdle. A 45° cephalic tilt view of the clavicle helps delineate further the degree of displacement and comminution at the fracture site and profiles the clavicle superior to the thorax. Particularly in high-energy or poly-traumatic injuries, a careful radiologic assessment of the shoulder girdle is essential to rule out any associated scapular or glenoid fractures [40]. In this scenario, a routine anteroposterior chest radiograph also is necessary to screen for associated rib fractures or intrathoracic injuries such as pneumothorax or hemothorax. An axillary view may become particularly useful in identifying subtle injuries to the lateral third of the clavicle. The serendipity view is a 40° cephalic tilt view coned over the SC joints that allows comparison of the bilateral SC joints to evaluate fractures and/or dislocations involving the medial third of the clavicle.

CT scanning is of little diagnostic value in an acute clavicle injury, except to rule out neurovascular and visceral injuries in the selected setting of an associated intra-articular glenoid fracture or a significantly displaced fracture-dislocation at the SC joint. It is more useful in evaluating the delayed union or non-union of a clavicle fracture. A CT angiogram or standard angiogram can be valuable in the setting of a distal vascular deficit following a clavicle fracture.

Management

The aim of clavicle fracture treatment is to reconstitute the clavicle as a rigid strut for the shoulder girdle to allow painless motion and strength around the shoulder while avoiding symptomatic non-union or malunion. Whenever possible, the least invasive means to accomplish this in each patient in a timely fashion should be the goal. In general, nonoperative treatment is preferred, and operative fixation for clavicle fracture have been reserved for open fractures, impending open fractures, associated neurovascular injuries, post-neurovascular repairs, floating shoulders, scapulothoracic dissociations, and fractures with polytrauma. Steady improvements in surgical technique and implant technology combined with the emergence of both objective and patient-based outcome studies with higher levels of evidence have challenged the notion that a good outcome can be obtained universally without operative management, however. The following sections present an evidence-based review of the literature regarding management of clavicle fractures and floating shoulders.

Fractures of the medial third of the clavicle

The medial third is the least commonly injured segment of the clavicle; less than 3% of all clavicle fractures involved this segment [2–8]. More recently, over a 5-year period at their tertiary trauma center, Throckmorton and colleagues [41] found the incidence of injuries to the medial third of the clavicle to be as high as 9.3% of all clavicle fractures. The key findings in this retrospective review of 57 fractures of the medial third of the clavicle highlighted the unique clinical features associated with these injuries. The major cause of injuries to the medial third of the clavicle was high-energy trauma: 84% of the patients were involved in motor vehicle collisions, and 90% had multisystem trauma. These fractures are difficult to visualize on plain radiographs and are best delineated with a CT scan (Fig. 3). This trend is consistent with the findings in the series by Postacchini and colleagues [4]. Associated intrathoracic injuries such as pneumo/hemothorax and lung contusions, as well as head and neck injuries, were found frequently. Overall, 93% of the patients were treated nonoperatively.

A number of authors have advocated nonoperative treatment of fractures of the medial third of the clavicle [3,11,15,36,39,41–43]. Given the relative paucity of these injuries, the literature on this topic is dominated by retrospective reviews with small sample sizes and by case reports. Moreover, confounding factors such as severe

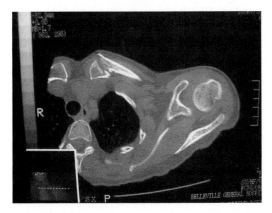

Fig. 3. Medial fractures of the clavicle are difficult to see on plain radiographs. CT scanning is the preferred imaging study for these injuries.

neurovascular or visceral injuries in polytrauma scenarios complicate the analysis of overall clinical outcome with or without operative treatment. Nevertheless, with the current level of evidence, nonoperative treatment with a period of immobilization is standard for most injuries of the medial third of the clavicle.

In selected clinical settings, however, operative treatments have been described and recommended [44–49]. Particularly in pediatric and adolescent patients, retrosternal SC dislocations or medial epiphyseal separations threatening the neck or the mediastinal contents often have been treated operatively [45–47]. In case reports, bipolar clavicle fractures, rare segmental fractures involving both the medial and lateral thirds of the clavicle, also have been deemed quite unstable and have been treated operatively with plates or screw fixation [48,49].

Fractures of the middle third of the clavicle

Fractures of the middle third of the clavicle are the most common type of clavicle fracture. The traditional view of nonoperative treatment of this type of fracture, irrespective of fracture characteristics or patient demographics, has been influenced principally by Neer's [50] series in 1960. In his review of 2235 patients who had nonoperatively treated fractures of the middle third of the clavicle, the non-union rate was 0.13%, compared with 4.6% in 45 patients treated operatively. A smaller review by Rowe [3] validated the notion, with non-union rates of 0.8% in patients treated nonoperatively and 3.7% in patients who received operative treatment. Given these findings, nonoperative treatment was recommended.

More than 200 different methods of immobilization, bracing, or sling treatments have been devised for the nonoperative treatment of displaced fractures of the clavicle. The number of treatments attests to the extreme difficulty of achieving and maintaining reduction [2,51]. Much of the effort spent in developing different ways of immobilizing the injured clavicle has been made against the near impossibility of maintaining the reduction and the impracticality of patient compliance [13,52–54]. As expected, no single superior method of immobilization has been found in any series [13,53–55]. A randomized study comparing a figure-of-eight brace versus a sling conducted by Andersen and colleagues [55] showed that there were no statistically significant functional or radiographic differences between the two groups. The brace was ineffective in restoring the bony alignment, and patients experienced difficulty tolerating the brace, clearly favoring the sling treatment. Moreover, there is no consensus on the optimal duration of immobilization or on the rehabilitation protocol for these injuries. Recommended periods of immobilization vary from 2 to 6 weeks, individualized to the patient's comfort level [13,53–56]. In addition, most authors recommend avoiding contact sports or heavy lifting for 4 to 6 months from the initial injury. Although good clinical outcomes can be achieved following nonoperative treatment, even after significant radiographic malunion, the rate of unsatisfactory outcomes increases with increasing fracture displacement [2,3,50,54,55,57]. The basic treatment protocol of immobilization as tolerated for 2 to 6 weeks followed by an individualized shoulder rehabilitation program as needed is an effective treatment modality for non- or minimally displaced fractures of the middle third of the clavicle.

A number of modern studies reporting a significant number of dissatisfied patients have emerged [7,53,58–61], challenging three facets of conventional wisdom concerning clavicle fractures: that the non-union rate is less than 1% with nonoperative treatment, that malunions cause functional deficit, and that operative treatment offers lower rates of non-union, symptomatic malunion and greater functional improvement in selected patients. Hill and colleagues [53] were one of the first groups to report a much higher-than-expected non-union rate following nonoperative treatment of fractures of the middle third of the clavicle. They reviewed 52 displaced clavicle fractures and found a non-union rate of 15% and a patient dissatisfaction rate of 31%, whereas in the older studies had lower rates of non-union [3,50]. Additionally, the study found that clavicle shortening of more than 2 cm was associated with lower patient satisfaction. Wick and colleagues [57], reviewing 33 delayed unions in fractures of the middle third of the clavicle, also found that more than 90% of them had more than 2 cm of shortening. A large, prospective observational study by Robinson and colleagues [7] analyzing 581 consecutive fractures of the middle third of the clavicle found an overall non-union rate of 4.5% at 6 months; the rate escalated to more than 20% in the subgroup that had displaced and comminuted fractures. The study also identified independent risk factors for non-

union, which included 100% displacement, fracture comminution, advanced age, and female gender. In their prospective study, Nowak and colleagues [58] also reported a non-union rate of 7% and similar risk factors for non-union. A recent systematic review of 2144 clavicle fractures validated these findings with a non-union rate of 15.1% in nonoperatively treated displaced fractures of the middle third of the clavicle [59]. Clearly, the rate of non-union with nonoperative treatment is not as low as previously estimated. Demographic differences between the older and the contemporary studies may play a significant role in the observed increase in non-union rates. As mentioned earlier, an increasing proportion of clavicle injuries reported in contemporary studies are caused by high-energy trauma or polytrauma [4–7,9,57,58]. These injuries are more likely to produce fracture patterns of increasing comminution and displacement, which are reported risk factors for non-union and poor outcomes [7,53,57–59].

As previously discussed, nonoperative treatment is quite ineffective in obtaining and maintaining an anatomic reduction of displaced clavicle fractures, so that radiographic malunion is ubiquitous. Clinical features such as shoulder weakness and easy fatigability with ptosis and/or scapular winging and thoracic outlet syndrome have been noted in the past [14,17,18,60,61]. This presentation is secondary to the typical displacement of the lateral (distal) fragment with inferior and medial translation and anterior rotation [14]. More recent studies estimated symptomatic malunion rates to be as high as 18% to 35% in nonoperatively treated patients [52,58,61]. An association between significant shortening (> 15–20 mm) of the clavicle and symptomatic malunion also has been reported in other studies [20,53,56,61]. In many established cases, restoration of the clavicle length by a corrective osteotomy improved patient-based outcome scores after symptomatic malunion [14,16–18]. To date, however, only two studies have showed statistically and clinically significant deficits in shoulder strength from clavicle shortening greater than 15 mm [20,62].

The non-union rate associated with operative treatment had been based on two widely cited older studies by Neer [50] and Rowe [3] (Fig. 4). Numerous recent retrospective series of operative fixation for acute fractures of the middle third of the clavicle reported pooled non-union rates well below 5%, however [63–73]. A recent systematic

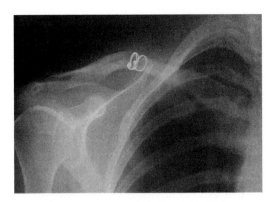

Fig. 4. In the past, operative treatment of clavicle fractures was plagued by inadequate fixation with high rates of delayed and non-union. Cerclage wiring alone is inherently unstable in the treatment of these injuries.

review of 460 displaced fractures of the middle third of the clavicle treated by plating had an overall non-union rate of 2.2% compared with a non-union rate of 15.1% in 159 similar fractures treated nonoperatively [59]. Similarly, a recent multicenter, randomized clinical trial by the Canadian Orthopaedic Trauma Society [52] comparing plate fixation versus sling treatment of displaced fractures of the middle third of the clavicle showed a significantly lower rate of non-union and symptomatic malunion in the surgical group. The trial also revealed that both surgeon-based and patient-based scores were significantly improved at all points of follow-up in the operated group. Improved surgical technique and implant designs and the judicious use of prophylactic antibiotics have contributed to improved overall surgical outcomes.

Primarily, two widely accepted methods of fixation—plate fixation or intramedullary pinning—are used in the operative treatment of fractures of the middle third of the clavicle. Any decision to treat fractures of the middle third of the clavicle operatively rather than nonoperatively must prompt a careful consideration of the advantages and the disadvantages of the treatment options. After carefully considering the risk factors for non-union and symptomatic malunion likely to cause functional impairments in an appropriate surgical candidate, one must take into consideration the possible complications inherent in operative treatment. These complications include deep or superficial wound infection, hardware-related irritation, hardware failure or migration, and poor cosmesis of a surgical scar. The data

reported in more recent clinical series show a universal decline in the rate of these complications, probably resulting from improved surgical technique and implant technology [63–74]. The timing of the chosen surgical intervention also may be an issue, because a recent retrospective study by Potter and colleagues [75] demonstrated a subtle decline in shoulder endurance strength and outcome measures with delayed plate fixation of clavicle malunion or non-union when compared with early fixation.

For plate fixation, dynamic compression plates, pelvic reconstruction plates, and anatomic precontoured plates have been used [12,63–69]. Although their low profile may lead to less skin irritation, semitubular plates and mini-plates were found to be mechanically too weak for rigid fixation and are not recommended [63,76,77]. Rigid plate fixation allows compression across the main fracture line combined with the use of interfragmentary compression screws as necessary. Plate fixation has superior biomechanical strength that offers excellent rotational and length control and allows early weight bearing on the limb. The main disadvantages are the long skin incision and tissue dissection around the fracture, the hardware prominence which may require plate removal, and possible refracture after the plate removal. As experience with precontoured "anatomic" plates and surgical technique increases, minimally invasive soft tissue handling can result in dramatic decreases in incision size. At present, there is no well-designed prospective study directly comparing clinical outcomes with different plate types. Intramedullary fixation with various devices including Kirschner wires, pins, rods, and screws also has been used widely [70–74]. Intramedullary fixation offers the advantages of being a soft tissue friendly and a minimally invasive or percutaneous procedure with the potential for improved cosmesis. The main disadvantages of this method of fixation (common to all "unlocked" intramedullary devices) are its inferior axial and rotational stability in nontransverse and comminuted fractures. Also, there have been reports of catastrophic migration of these implants—specifically smooth pins—elsewhere in the body [78–80]. Again, no comparative studies evaluating different types of intramedullary devices or of plates versus intramedullary fixation are available. Clearly, these voids in higher-level evidence regarding the operative treatment of fractures of the middle third of the clavicle need to be filled through future studies.

Operative technique

Currently, the senior author's preferred operative treatment for displaced fractures of the middle third of the clavicle is rigid fixation using anatomically precontoured 3.5-mm dynamic compression plates combined with interfragmentary compression screws as needed (Figs. 5 and 6). Operative treatment is recommended for patients who have traditional indications (eg, open fractures, neurovascular compromise) and for young, active individuals who have completely displaced fractures, obvious deformity, and shortening of 1.5 to 2.0 cm or greater displacement. A detailed surgical technique has been published recently and is similar to that used for fractures of the lateral third of the clavicle [81]. The plate usually is placed on the superior aspect of the clavicle, because this placement has been shown to be the most advantageous biomechanically. As familiarity with the technique improves, smaller skin incisions, extensive mobilization of subcutaneous tissue, and other minimally invasive techniques can be used to decrease soft tissue stripping and dissection. Whenever possible, branches of the supraclavicular nerves are identified, mobilized, and protected. A minimum of three bicortical screws are used distal and proximal to the fracture; a lag screw is placed whenever possible. Smaller fracture fragments (including a fairly consistent vertically oriented anterior cortical fragment) are "teased" into position without stripping all their soft tissue. They can be fixed with small or mini-fragment screws or sutured into place. Because this procedure typically is reserved for young, active patients, bone quality rarely is an issue, and the authors have not found locking plates to be required or useful in this setting. It is important to perform a two-layer closure of the soft tissue to maximize local resistance to infection and to minimize the potential for hardware irritation. The myofascial layer is sutured with #1 absorbable suture, followed by #2-0 subcutaneous sutures and clips for the skin. The patient wears a simple sling for comfort and can begin range-of-motion exercises immediately. The use of the sling is discontinued at 10 to 14 days, and strengthening exercises are initiated at 6 weeks. Full-contact activities usually are restricted for 12 weeks, but patient compliance with this restriction is highly variable.

Fractures of the lateral third of the clavicle

Most fractures of the lateral third of the clavicle (especially fractures that are non- or minimally displaced) can be treated successfully with a period of immobilization. A certain proportion of the fractures involving the lateral third of the clavicle are significantly displaced, however, and are at high risk for delayed or non-union. In Neer's [50] original series of clavicle fractures, he observed the unusually high rate of non-union in displaced fractures of the lateral third of the clavicle. The fractures he later classified as type II, in which the fracture occurs medial to the CC ligaments and hence is detached from the displaced medial fragment, had a particularly high rate of delayed union or non-union [37]. In type II fractures, which are much less common than the undisplaced type I injury, he recommended operative stabilization. Later series reported similar rates of non-union ranging from 22% to 33%, and several authors recommended operative treatment of displaced fractures of the lateral third of the clavicle [82–88]. Three contemporary studies have reported estimated non-union rates ranging from 22% to 37% for these injuries treated non-operatively, validating the findings of previous studies [7,89,90]. Interestingly, two of these studies also found that a large proportion of the non-united fractures were asymptomatic, usually in elderly, sedentary individuals [89,90]. The

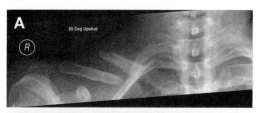
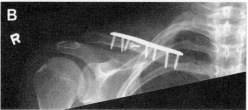

Fig. 5. (*A*) A displaced mid-shaft clavicle fracture with significant shortening. This degree of shortening is an indication for primary operative fixation in a healthy, young, active individual. (*B*) After fixation with an anatomic clavicle plate, solid bony union in an anatomic position was achieved, with rapid restoration of normal shoulder function.

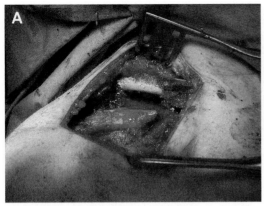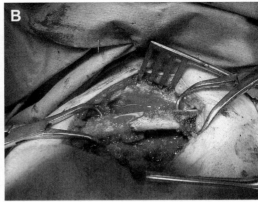

Fig. 6. (*A*) Intraoperatively, the fracture site is exposed and debrided. (*B*) Reduction is performed with the aid of reduction forceps or towel clips. Typically, little force is required for reduction, and it rarely is necessary to free drape the arm.

long-term (mean, 15 years) follow-up study by Nordqvist and colleagues [89] reviewing 110 fractures of the lateral third of the clavicle treated nonoperatively showed that eight of the their non-union cases had no significant deficits based on patient-based outcome measures. In Robinson's [90] series of 101 patients who had nonoperatively treated fractures of the lateral third of the clavicle, there were no statistically significant differences in Constant and Short Form-36 scores between those with and without non-union or between those with and without delayed operative fixation. Twenty-one of the 32 cases of non-union (66%) also were deemed by the patients to be asymptomatic enough to avoid delayed surgical treatment at an average follow-up of 6.2 years. Still to be determined through prospective prognostic studies are possible radiologic and/or clinical risk factors for symptomatic non-union to help guide timely, active treatment.

There are no prospective studies comparing operative versus nonoperative treatment for fractures of the lateral third of the clavicle. In terms of methods of fixation, the orthopedic literature is dominated by small case series based on an array of different technical variations using wires, screws, pins, and plates [37,83,84,86,87,91–100]. These methods include open and arthroscopic combinations of transacromial stabilization using Kirschner wires, tension banding, transacromial screws or pins, plates, CC screw fixation, CC ligament reconstruction or repair, and subcoracoid "slings." Only one study directly compared two different methods of operative fixation: Flinkkila and colleagues [93] retrospectively compared Kirschner wire fixation versus hook plating and

showed the use of the transacromial wire to be fraught with complications such as infections, wire breakage, and wire migration. These complications previously had been reported [101]. Interest in the use of the hook plate (with a smooth, subacromial extension of the plate to maintain position of the distal clavicular fragment) to treat these injuries has increased recently because the plate's stable anatomic and biomechanical properties allow early shoulder mobilization and weight bearing. The high incidence of subacromial impingement and shoulder stiffness often necessitates removal of the plate, however [91–93]. Resection of the distal clavicle has little role in the setting of an acute fracture; however, intra-articular fractures (Neer type III) involving the AC joint eventually may cause a posttraumatic arthritis of the joint that is amenable to such intervention [102].

In summary, most fractures of the lateral third of the clavicle should be treated nonoperatively. Even though non-union does occur frequently with displaced (Neer type II) fractures of the lateral third of the clavicle, recent clinical studies suggest that many non-unions in elderly, sedentary individuals are asymptomatic. Given the current paucity of high-level therapeutic evidence regarding these injuries, operative treatment should be individualized and reserved for young, active patients (especially those engaged in throwing or overhead activity) who have completely displaced fractures of the distal clavicle. Further prospective studies are needed to optimize the approach and treatment modalities for managing fractures of the lateral third of the clavicle.

Operative technique

Currently, the senior author's treatment of choice for displaced fractures of the lateral third of the clavicle is to employ rigid fixation using either anatomically precontoured distal clavicular plates or hook plates.

The patient is placed in the beach-chair position with the head secured on a headrest. The shoulder is prepped and draped to include the SC joint; the authors do not free drape the arm routinely. The AC joint and the fracture site are palpated to determine the center of the skin incision. An oblique skin incision is made over the fracture on the superior border of the clavicle and is extended across the AC joint. A single, thick layer of subcutaneous tissue flap is raised, exposing the underlying myofascial layer. This layer then is divided sharply down to the clavicle and is elevated off the bone as a single layer to cover the plate later. The fracture site then is exposed and inspected. After the fracture hematoma and interposed soft tissue are debrided, bone-holding forceps are used for anatomic reduction of the fracture. If a low-profile "anatomic" plate is used for fixation, the plate first can be fixed provisionally to the medial-clavicle fragment to aid in reduction. Anatomic distal clavicle plates offer extra holes for screws in the cancellous bone of the distal clavicle to enhance distal fixation (Fig. 7). It rarely is necessary to cross the AC joint for fixation: if required, unicortical screws can be used to avoid impinging on the subacromial space. If a hook plate is used, a cautery is used to create an opening posterior to the AC joint to pass the hook underneath the acromion before setting the plate down onto the reduced clavicle. One must be careful not to cauterize deep into the subacromial space, because doing so may damage the rotator cuff muscles and cause excessive bleeding from the subacromial bursa. Screws are inserted into the plate, taking care not to violate the subclavicular space. In selected cases, with a very small distal fragment, hook plate fixation can be supplemented with the modified Weaver-Dunn procedure. This procedure involves mobilization of a wafer of bone along with the coracoacromial ligament from the acromion. The bony wafer is attached into or onto the distal end of the clavicle with a nonabsorbable suture (Fig. 8).

Once the internal fixation is complete, the wound is irrigated thoroughly and is closed in two layers. Closure of the deeper myofascial layer

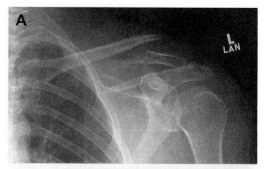

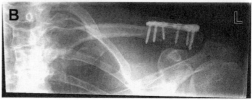

Fig. 7. (*A*) A displaced fracture of the lateral third of the clavicle after a cycling accident in a young, active individual. (*B*) Plate fixation resulted in rapid union in an anatomic position.

is very important to cover the plate and minimize problems with prominent hardware later. The incision then is infiltrated with 0.5% bupivacaine solution for postoperative pain control, and the arm is placed into a sling.

Postoperatively, the arm stays in the sling on a full-time basis for 2 weeks followed by active assistive range-of-motion exercises in the scapular plane of motion. Full active range-of-motion exercises are begun at 4 weeks followed by strengthening of the shoulder girdle at 6 to 8 weeks. Return to sports can be considered 3 months after surgery.

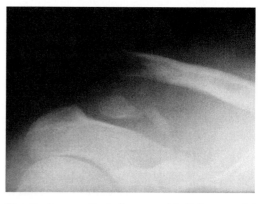

Fig. 8. A very distal fracture with little potential purchase in the distal fragment is a relative indication to augment fixation with a hook plate or coracoclavicular screw if operative intervention is chosen.

Floating shoulder

Floating shoulder is a rare injury pattern consisting of ipsilateral clavicle and glenoid neck fractures. This injury initially was considered inherently unstable, because the glenoid loses both osseous and ligamentous contact with the scapula and the clavicle. The perceived concern was that the weight of the arm and the pull of the muscles around the shoulder girdle continue to displace the glenohumeral joint inferiorly as well as anteromedially. In a cadaver study, Williams and colleagues [103] performed sequential osseous and ligamentous sectioning around the AC joint and found that fractures of the clavicle and the scapula must be accompanied by ligament disruptions to result in a floating shoulder.

Given the combined injuries to the stabilizers of the shoulder suspensory complex, early reports recommended operative management to restore stability to the shoulder girdle [104,105]. The authors reported good to excellent outcomes in most patients who had operative fixation of the clavicle and/or the glenoid. Edwards and colleagues [106] reported a retrospective review of 20 patients treated nonoperatively for floating shoulders. Nineteen of the 20 patients reported good to excellent results, especially when fracture displacement was less than 5 mm. Further studies retrospectively comparing operative and nonoperative treatment groups showed no significant differences between the two groups in radiologic or functional outcome measures [107–109]. The authors' general consensus was that operative fixation could be considered for significantly displaced fractures but that an individualized approach to treatment was more important.

To date, all the studies regarding treatment of floating shoulders are retrospective reviews limited by small patient numbers and surgeons' bias. Because of the rarity of this injury pattern, it will be challenging to generate enough number of cases to compare therapy modalities in a prospective manner. For now, the authors recommend the moderate approach of treating each injury individually and managing operatively any symptomatic or grossly unstable injury patterns based on radiographs and clinical examinations.

Summary

Clavicle fractures are one of the most common upper extremity injuries encountered in orthopedic practice. In most cases, rare fractures involving the medial third of the clavicle are treated adequately with a period of immobilization, particularly in an isolated setting. Given the incidence of associated injuries, a careful diagnostic evaluation is important. There is increasing evidence supporting primary operative fixation of completely displaced mid-shaft fractures of the clavicle, especially in young, active patients who have visible deformity or shortening of 1.5 to 2.0 cm or more. Although a number of fixation methods are available, none has been proven to be definitively superior to the others. At present, an anatomic, precontoured compression plate placed on the superior aspect of the bone through a minimally invasive approach is the authors' preferred operative treatment. Completely displaced fractures of the lateral third of the clavicle respond well to nonoperative treatment but have a high rate of delayed and non-union. This failure to achieve union may produce minimal symptomatology in older, sedentary individuals; primary operative repair should be considered in younger individuals, especially those who perform overhead activities regularly. A floating shoulder is a rare clinical entity that has been treated both operatively and nonoperatively with good clinical outcomes in the past. Therapy recommendations cannot be made with the current level of evidence, and thus treatment must be individualized, usually based on the degree of displacement: greater deformity and a higher activity levels are indications for more aggressive primary treatment. Further well-designed prospective and randomized, controlled trials are needed to provide further insights into the evolving management of this common orthopedic injury.

References

[1] Adams F. The genuine works of Hippocrates. New York: William Wood; 1886.

[2] Neer CS. Fractures of the clavicle. In: Rockwood CA Jr, Green DP, editors. Fractures in adults. 2nd edition. Philadelphia: JB Lippincott Company; 1984. p. 707–13.

[3] Rowe CR. An atlas of anatomy and treatment of mid-clavicular fractures. Clin Orthop 1968;58: 29–42.

[4] Postacchini F, Gumina S, De Santis P, et al. Epidemiology of clavicle fractures. J Shoulder Elbow Surg 2002;11:454–6.

[5] Nordqvist A, Petersson C. The incidence of fractures of the clavicle. Clin Orthop 1994;300:127–32.

[6] Robinson CM. Fractures of the clavicle in the adult: epidemiology and classification. J Bone Joint Surg Br 1998;80:476–84.

[7] Robinson CM, Court-Brown CM, McQueen MM, et al. Estimating the risk of nonunion following nonoperative treatment of a clavicular fracture. J Bone Joint Surg Am 2004;86(7):1359–65.

[8] Nowak J, Mallmin H, Larsson S. The aetiology and epidemiology of clavicular fractures: a prospective study during a two-year period in Uppsala, Sweden. Injury 2000;31:353–8.

[9] McKee MD, Schemitsch EH, Stephen DJ, et al. Functional outcome following clavicle fractures in polytrauma patient [abstract]. J Trauma 1999;47:616.

[10] Gardner E. The embryology of the clavicle. Clin Orthop 1968;58:9–16.

[11] Lewonowski K, Bassett GS. Complete posterior sternoclavicular epiphyseal separation. A case report and review of the literature. Clin Orthop 1992;281:84–8.

[12] Huang JI, Toogood P, Chen MR, et al. Clavicular anatomy and the applicability of precontoured plates. J Bone Joint Surg Am 2007;89:2260–5.

[13] Lazarus MD. Fractures of the clavicle. In: Bucholz RW, Heckman JD, editors. Rockwood and Green's fractures in adults. 5th edition. Philadelphia: Lippincott Williams & Wilkins; 2002. p. 1041–78.

[14] McKee MD, Wild LM, Schemitsch EH. Midshaft malunions of the clavicle. J Bone Joint Surg Am 2003;85:790–7.

[15] Jupiter JB, Ring D. Fractures of the clavicle. In: Iannotti JP, Williams GR, editors. Disorders of the shoulder: diagnosis and management. Philadelphia: Lippincott Williams & Wilkins; 1999. p. 709–36.

[16] Basamania CJ. Claviculoplasty. J Shoulder Elbow Surg 1999;8(5):540.

[17] Bosch U, Skutek M, Peters G, et al. Extension osteotomy in malunited clavicular fractures. J Shoulder Elbow Surg 1998;7(4):402–5.

[18] Chan KY, Jupiter JB, Leffert RD, et al. Clavicle malunion. J Shoulder Elbow Surg 1999;8(4):287–90.

[19] Kuhne JE. Symptomatic malunions of the middle clavicle [abstract]. J Shoulder Elbow Surg 1999;8(5):539.

[20] McKee MD, Pedersen EM, Jones C, et al. Deficits following non-operative treatment of displaced, mid-shaft clavicle fractures. J Bone Joint Surg Am 2006;88:35–40.

[21] Rumball KM, Da Silva VF, Preston DN, et al. Brachial plexus injury after clavicular fracture: case report and literature review. Can J Surg 1991;34:264–6.

[22] Lange RH, Noel SH. Traumatic lateral scapular displacement: an expanded spectrum of associated neurovascular injury. J Orthop Trauma 1993;7:361–6.

[23] Katras T, Baltazar U, Rush DS, et al. Subclavian arterial injury associated with blunt trauma. Vasc Surg 2001;35(1):43–50.

[24] Kendall KM, Burton JH, Cushing B. Fatal subclavian artery transection from isolated clavicle fracture. J Trauma 2000;48(2):316–8.

[25] Barbier O, Malghem J, Delaere O, et al. Injury to the brachial plexus by a fragment of bone after fracture of the clavicle. J Bone Joint Surg Br 1997;79:534–6.

[26] Simpson NS, Jupiter JB. Clavicular nonunion and malunion: evaluation and surgical management. J Am Acad Orthop Surg 1996;4:1–8.

[27] Ludewig PM, Behrens SA, Meyer SM, et al. Three-dimensional clavicular motion during arm elevation: reliability and descriptive data. J Orthop Sports Phys Ther 2004;34:140–9.

[28] Andermahr J, Jubel A, Elsner A, et al. Malunion of the clavicle causes significant glenoid malposition: a quantitative anatomic investigation. Surg Radiol Anat 2006;28(5):447–56.

[29] Stanley D, Trowbridge EA, Norris SH. The mechanism of clavicular fracture: a clinical and biomechanical analysis. J Bone Joint Surg Br 1988;70:461–4.

[30] Ebraheim NA, An HS, Jackson WT, et al. Scapulothoracic dissociation. J Bone Joint Surg Am 1988;70 428.

[31] Spar I. Total claviculectomy for pathological fractures. Clin Orthop 1977;129:236–7.

[32] Bernard RN Jr, Haddad RJ Jr. Enchondroma of the proximal clavicle. An unusual cause of pathologic fracture-dislocaition of the sternoclavicular joint. Clin Orthop 1982;167:239–41.

[33] To EW, Pang PC, Tsang WS, et al. Pathologic fracture of clavicle after radiotherapy. Am J Roentgenol 2001;176(1):264–5.

[34] Fallon KE, Fricker PA. Stress fracture of the clavicle in a young female gymnast. Br J Sports Med 2001;35(6):448–9.

[35] Wu CD, Chen YC. Stress fracture of the clavicle in a professional baseball player. J Shoulder Elbow Surg 1998;7(2):164–7.

[36] Allman FL Jr. Fractures and ligamentous injuries of the clavicle and its articulation. J Bone Joint Surg Am 1967;49:774–84.

[37] Neer CS. Fractures of the distal third of the clavicle. Clin Orthop 1968;58:43–50.

[38] Rockwood CA. Fractures of the outer clavicle in children and adults. J Bone Joint Surg Br 1982;64:642–7.

[39] Craig EV. Fractures of the clavicle. In: Rockwood CA, Matsen FA, editors. The shoulder. Philadelphia: WB Saunders; 1990. p. 367–412.

[40] DeFranco MJ, Patterson BM. The floating shoulder. J Am Acad Orthop Surg 2006;14(8):499–509.

[41] Throckmorton T, Kuhn JE. Fractures of the medial end of the clavicle. J Shoulder Elbow Surg 2007;16(1):49–54.

[42] Zaslav KR, Ray S, Neer CS. Conservative management of a displaced medial clavicular physeal injury in an adolescent athlete. A case report and literature review. Am J Sports Med 1989;17: 833–6.

[43] Herscovici D Jr, Sanders R, DiPasquale T, et al. Injuries of the shoulder girdle. Clin Orthop 1995;318: 54–60.

[44] Brinker MR, Bartz RL, Reardon PR, et al. A method for open reduction and internal fixation of the unstable posterior sternoclavicular joint dislocation. J Orthop Trauma 1997;11(5):378–81.

[45] Waters PM, Bae DS, Kadiyala RK. Short-term outcomes after surgical treatment of traumatic posterior sternoclavicular fracture-dislocations in children and adolescents. J Ped Orthop 2003; 23(4):464–9.

[46] Yang J, al-Etani H, Letts M. Diagnosis and treatment of posterior sternoclavicular joint dislocations in children. Am J Orthop 1996;25(8):565–9.

[47] Goldfarb CA, Bassett GS, Sullivan S, et al. Retrosternal displacement after physeal fracture of the medial clavicle in children treatment by open reduction and internal fixation. J Bone Joint Surg Br 2001;83(8):1168–72.

[48] Wade AM, Barrett MO, Crist BD, et al. Medial clavicular epiphyseal fracture with ipsilateral acromio—clavicular dislocation: a case report of panclavicular fracture dislocation. J Orthop Trauma 2007;21(6):418–21.

[49] Pang KP, Yung SW, Lee TS, et al. Bipolar clavicular injury. Med J Malaysia 2003;58(4):621–4.

[50] Neer CS. Nonunion of the clavicle. JAMA 1972; 1960:1006–11.

[51] Crenshaw AH Jr. Fractures of the shoulder girdle, arm and forearm. In: Crenshaw AH Jr, editor. Campbell's operative orthopaedics, 8th edition. St. Louis: Mosby-Yearbook Inc.; 1992. p. 989–95.

[52] Canadian Orthopaedic Trauma Society. Nonoperative treatment compared with plate fixation of displaced midshaft clavicular fractures: a multi-center, randomized clinical trial. J Bone Joint Surg Am 2007;89:1–10.

[53] Hill JM, McGuire MH, Crosby LA. Closed treatment of displaced middle-third fractures of the clavicle gives poor results. J Bone Joint Surg Br 1997;79:537–9.

[54] Nordqvist A, Petersson CJ, Redlund-Johnell I. Mid-clavicle fractures in adults: end result study after conservative treatment. J Orthop Trauma 1998; 12:572–6.

[55] Andersen K, Jensen PO, Lauritzen J. Treatment of clavicular fractures: figure-of-eight versus a simple sling. Acta Orthop Scand 1987;58:71–4.

[56] Eskola A, Vainionpaa S, Myllynen P, et al. Outcome of clavicular fracture in 89 patients. Arch Orthop Trauma Surg 1986;105:337–8.

[57] Wick M, Müller EJ, Kollig E, et al. Midshaft fractures of the clavicle with a shortening of more than

2 cm predispose to nonunion. Arch Orthop Trauma Surg 2001;121(4):207–11.

[58] Nowak J, Holgersson M, Larsson S. Sequelae from clavicular fractures are common: a prospective study of 222 patients. Acta Orthop 2005;76(4): 496–502.

[59] Zlowodzki M, Zelle BA, Cole PA, et al. Treatment of acute midshaft clavicle fractures: systematic review of 2144 fractures: on behalf of the Evidence-Based Orthopaedic Trauma Working Group. J Orthop Trauma 2005;19(7):504–7.

[60] Kuhne JE. Symptomatic malunions of the middle clavicle. J Shoulder Elbow Surg 1999;8(5):539.

[61] Lazarides S, Zafiropoulos G. Conservative treatment of fractures at the middle third of the clavicle: the relevance of shortening and clinical outcome. J Shoulder Elbow Surg 2006;15(2):191–4.

[62] Ledger M, Leeks N, Ackland T, et al. Short malunions of the clavicle: an anatomic and functional study. J Shoulder Elbow Surg 2005;14:349–54.

[63] Poigenfurst J, Rappold G, Fischer W. Plating of fresh clavicular fractures: results of 122 operations. Injury 1992;23:237–41.

[64] McKee MD, Seiler JG, Jupiter JB. The application of the limited contact dynamic compression plate in the upper extremity: an analysis of 114 consecutive cases. Injury 1995;26(10):661–6.

[65] Russo R, Visconti V, Lorini S, et al. Displaced comminuted midshaft clavicle fractures: use of Mennen plate fixation system. J Trauma 2007; 63(4):951–4.

[66] Shen WJ, Liu TJ, Shen YS. Plate fixation of fresh displaced midshaft clavicle fractures. Injury 1999; 30(7):497–500.

[67] Collinge C, Devinney S, Herscovici D, et al. Anterior-inferior plate fixation of middle-third fractures and nonunions of the clavicle. J Orthop Trauma 2006;20(10):680–6.

[68] Shahid R, Mushtaq A, Maqsood M. Plate fixation of clavicle fractures: a comparative study between reconstruction plate and dynamic compression plate. Acta Orthop Belg 2007;73(2):170–4.

[69] Coupe BD, Wimhurst JA, Indar R, et al. A new approach for plate fixation of midshaft clavicular fractures. Injury 2005;36(10):1166–71.

[70] Jubel A, Andermahr J, Schiffer G, et al. Elastic stable intramedullary nailing of midclavicular fractures with a titanium nail. Clin Orthop 2003;408: 279–85.

[71] Chu CM, Wang SJ, Lin LC. Fixation of mid-third clavicular fractures with Knowles pins: 78 patients followed for 2–7 years. Acta Orthop Scand 2002; 73(2):134–9.

[72] Chuang TY, Ho WP, Hsieh PH, et al. Closed reduction and internal fixation for acute midshaft clavicular fractures using cannulated screws. J Trauma 2006;60(6):1315–20.

[73] Kettler M, Schieker M, Braunstein V, et al. Flexible intramedullary nailing for stabilization of displaced

midshaft clavicle fractures: technique and results in 87 patients. Acta Orthop 2007;78(3):424–9, 79.

[74] Strauss EJ, Egol KA, France MA, et al. Complications of intramedullary Hagie pin fixation for acute midshaft clavicle fractures. J Shoulder Elbow Surg 2007;16(3):280–4.

[75] Potter JM, Jones C, Wild LM, et al. The restoration of objectively measured shoulder strength and patient-oriented outcome after immediate fixation versus delayed reconstruction of displaced midshaft fractures of the clavicle. J Shoulder Elbow Surg 2007;16(5):514–8.

[76] Böstman O, Manninen M, Pihlajamäki H. Complications of plate fixation in fresh displaced midclavicular fractures. J Trauma 1997;43(5):778–83.

[77] Schwarz N, Hocker K. Osteosynthesis of irreducible fractures of the clavicle with 2.7-mm ASIF plates. J Trauma 1992;33:179–83.

[78] Nordback I, Markkula H. Migration of Kirschner pin from the clavicle into the ascending aorta. Acta Chir Scand 1985;151:177–9.

[79] Maget R Jr. Migration of a Kirschner wire from the shoulder region into the lung: report of two cases. J Bone Joint Surg Am 1943;25:477–83.

[80] Lyons FA, Rockwood CA Jr. Migration of pins used in operations on the shoulder. J Bone Joint Surg Am 1990;72:1262–7.

[81] Altamimi SA, McKee MD, Canadian Orthopaedic Trauma Society. Nonoperative treatment compared with plate fixation of displaced midshaft clavicular fractures. Surgical technique. J Bone Joint Surg Am 2008;90(Suppl 2):1–8.

[82] Eskola A, Vainionpaa S, Patiala H, et al. Outcome of operative treatment in fresh lateral clavicular fracture. Ann Chir Gynaecol 1987;76:167–9.

[83] Edwards DJ, Kavanagh TG, Flannery MC. Fractures of the distal clavicle: a case for fixation. Injury 1992;23:44–6.

[84] Goldberg JA, Bruce WJ, Sonnabend DH, et al. Type 2 fractures of the distal clavicle: a new surgical technique. J Shoulder Elbow Surg 1997;6(4):380–2.

[85] Jupiter JB, Leffert RD. Nonunion of the clavicle. Associated complications and surgical management. J Bone Joint Surg Am 1987;69:753–60.

[86] Ballmer FT, Gerber C. Coracoclavicular screw fixation for unstable fractures of the distal clavicle. A report of five cases. J Bone Joint Surg Br 1991;73: 291–4.

[87] Yamaguchi H, Arakawa H, Kobayashi M. Results of the Bosworth method for unstable fractures of the distal clavicle. Int Orthop 1998;22(6):366–8.

[88] Deafenbaugh MK, Dugdale TW, Staeheli JW, et al. Nonoperative treatment of Neer type II distal clavicle fractures: a prospective study. Contemp Orthop 1990;20:405–13.

[89] Nordqvist A, Petersson C, Redlund-Johnell I. The natural course of lateral clavicle fracture. 15 (11-21) year follow-up of 110 cases. Acta Orthop Scand 1993;64:87–91.

[90] Robinson CM, Cairns DA. Primary nonoperative treatment of displaced lateral fractures of the clavicle. J Bone Joint Surg Am 2004;86(4): 778–82.

[91] Meda PV, Machani B, Sinopidis C, et al. Clavicular hook plate for lateral end fractures: a prospective study. Injury 2006;37(3):277–83.

[92] Kashii M, Inui H, Yamamoto K. Surgical treatment of distal clavicle fractures using the clavicular hook plate. Clin Orthop 2006;447:158–64.

[93] Flinkkilä T, Ristiniemi J, Hyvönen P, et al. Surgical treatment of unstable fractures of the distal clavicle: a comparative study of Kirschner wire and clavicular hook plate fixation. Acta Orthop Scand 2002;73(1):50–3.

[94] Scadden JE, Richards R. Intramedullary fixation of Neer type 2 fractures of the distal clavicle with an AO/ASIF screw. Injury 2005;36(10):1172–5.

[95] Nourissat G, Kakuda C, Dumontier C, et al. Arthroscopic stabilization of Neer type 2 fracture of the distal part of the clavicle. Arthroscopy 2007;23(6):674.e1–4.

[96] Chen CH, Chen WJ, Shih CH. Surgical treatment for distal clavicle fracture with coracoclavicular ligament disruption. J Trauma 2002;52(1):72–8.

[97] Jin CZ, Kim HK, Min BH. Surgical treatment for distal clavicle fracture associated with coracoclavicular ligament rupture using a cannulated screw fixation technique. J Trauma 2006;60(6): 1358–61.

[98] Badhe SP, Lawrence TM, Clark DI. Tension band suturing for the treatment of displaced type 2 lateral end clavicle fractures. Arch Orthop Trauma Surg 2007;127(1):25–8.

[99] Kao FC, Chao EK, Chen CH, et al. Treatment of distal clavicle fracture using Kirschner wires and tension-band wires. J Trauma 2001;51(3):522–5.

[100] Bezer M, Aydin N, Guven O. The treatment of distal clavicle fractures with coracoclavicular ligament disruption: a report of 10 cases. J Orthop Trauma 2005;19(8):524–8.

[101] Kona J, Bosse MJ, Staeheli JW, et al. Type II distal clavicle fractures: a retrospective review of surgical treatment. J Orthop Trauma 1990;4:115–20.

[102] Rabalais RD, McCarty E. Surgical treatment of symptomatic acromioclavicular joint problems: a systematic review. Clin Orthop 2007;455:30–7.

[103] Williams GR Jr, Naranja J, Klimkiewicz J, et al. The floating shoulder: a biomechanical basis for classification and management. J Bone Joint Surg Am 2001;83(8):1182–7.

[104] Leung KS, Lam TP. Open reduction and internal fixation of ipsilateral fractures of the scapular neck and clavicle. J Bone Joint Surg Am 1993; 75(7):1015–8.

[105] Herscovici D Jr, Fiennes AG, Allgöwer M, et al. The floating shoulder: ipsilateral clavicle and scapular neck fractures. J Bone Joint Surg Br 1992; 74(3):362–4.

[106] Edwards SG, Whittle AP, Wood GW II. Nonoperative treatment of ipsilateral fractures of the scapula and clavicle. J Bone Joint Surg Am 2000; 82(6):774–80.

[107] van Noort A, te Slaa RL, Marti RK, et al. The floating shoulder. A multicentre study. J Bone Joint Surg Br 2001;83(6):795–8.

[108] Egol KA, Connor PM, Karunakar MA, et al. The floating shoulder: clinical and functional results. J Bone Joint Surg Am 2001;83(8): 1188–94.

[109] Labler L, Platz A, Weishaupt D, et al. Clinical and functional results after floating shoulder injuries. J Trauma 2004;57(3):595–602.

ELSEVIER
SAUNDERS

Orthop Clin N Am 39 (2008) 507–518

ORTHOPEDIC
CLINICS
OF NORTH AMERICA

Anterior Glenohumeral Joint Dislocations

Christopher C. Dodson, MD, Frank A. Cordasco, MD*

*Sports Medicine and Shoulder Service, Hospital for Special Surgery, 535 East 70th Street,
New York, NY 10021, USA*

The glenohumeral joint is the most mobile articulation in the body and the most commonly dislocated diarthroidal joint. The incidence of shoulder dislocation is bimodal, with peaks occurring during the second and sixth decades of life [1,2]. Anterior dislocation is by far the most common direction and can lead to instability of the glenohumeral joint, which ranges from subtle increased laxity to recurrent dislocation.

Traumatic injury is the most common cause of shoulder instability, accounting for approximately 95% of anterior shoulder dislocations [1–4]. The sequela of traumatic anterior dislocation is related to the age of the patient at the time of initial dislocation and the degree of injury. The patients' age at the time of injury is inversely related to the recurrence rate. In patients younger than 20 years of age, recurrent dislocation rates have been reported as high as 90% in the athletic population. The rate of recurrence drops to between 50% and 75% in patients 20 to 25 years of age [1–4]. In patients older than 40 years, anterior dislocation is associated with lower rates of instability, but high rates of rotator cuff tears. The incidence of rotator cuff tears in patients older than 40 years at the time of initial dislocation is 15% and the incidence climbs to 40% in patients older than 60 years of age [1]. The recurrence rate is directly related to the degree of injury to the supporting structures of the shoulder at the time of the initial dislocation. The presence and size of the Bankart tear, the presence and size of osseous lesions including Hill-Sachs defects, osseous Bankart lesions, and glenoid bone loss, and finally

the degree of capsular and rotator cuff pathology all play a significant role [5–7].

Traditionally, anterior shoulder instability was treated using open techniques that were based on restoring the capsulolabral anatomy. Over time, understanding of anterior shoulder dislocations and the resulting instability has improved. Likewise, significant advances in arthroscopic equipment have allowed use of the arthroscope to address anatomically the various lesions that cause instability. The ideal patient for anterior surgical stabilization has clear unidirectional instability and has failed conservative management. Additionally, the ideal shoulder has a Bankart lesion with robust labral tissue for repair. The goal is to repair anatomically the capsulolabral injury and reduce the capsular volume to eliminate instability. Whether the procedure is done open or arthroscopically is irrelevant provided that it produces comparable clinical outcomes. It is important that whichever technique is chosen, the surgeon should be prepared to address all concomitant pathology that can be encountered in the patients' shoulder. This article reviews the anatomy, pathophysiology, clinical evaluation, and treatment of anterior shoulder instability. The recommendations regarding diagnosis and treatment presented in this article are based on the senior author's (FAC) clinical experience.

Anatomy and pathophysiology

The normal humeral head translates only 1 mm from the center of the glenoid during active motion [8,9]. The glenohumeral joint is stabilized by both dynamic and static restraints. The static stabilizers consist of the glenoid labrum, the

* Corresponding author.
E-mail address: cordascof@hss.edu (F.A. Cordasco).

articular surface of the glenoid, negative intra-articular pressure, and the capsuloligamentous structures. Dynamic stabilizers include the rotator cuff muscles (particularly the lower subscapularis); pectoralis major; latissimus dorsi; biceps; and periscapular musculature. In general, the capsular ligaments provide stability at end range of motion, whereas during midrange of motion, the capsuloligamentous structures are lax and the joint is stabilized by dynamic joint compression. Glenohumeral instability occurs when there is a deficiency in the bony, soft tissue, or dynamic muscular restraints to translation of the humeral head on the glenoid. Generally speaking, rehabilitation following instability episodes is directed toward optimizing the dynamic stabilizers, whereas surgical intervention restores the static stabilizers [10].

The oval glenoid is longest in its inferior-superior diameter and has a nearly flat articular surface. Although the osseous shape of the glenoid does not contribute greatly to stability, the chondral surface of the glenoid is thickened, creating a concave articular surface that improves glenohumeral stability. The labrum is a fibrous structure that is firmly attached to the glenoid at its inferior margin and bound more loosely superiorly where it is confluent with the origin of the long head of the biceps tendon. Howell and Galinat [11] demonstrated that the labrum contributes approximately 50% of the total depth of the socket. Furthermore, they noted that detachment of the labrum anteriorly, as in a Bankart lesion, may reduce the depth of the socket in the anteroposterior direction from approximately 5 mm to 2.4 mm. They likened the labrum to a "chock block" and concluded that the loss of the labrum is an important etiologic factor in anterior instability.

The ligaments of the glenohumeral joint are discrete bands that insert onto the glenoid labrum. The important ligaments are the superior glenohumeral ligament, the middle glenohumeral ligament, and the inferior glenohumeral ligament complex (Fig. 1). The superior glenohumeral ligament originates on the superoanterior rim of the glenoid, just anterior to the biceps origin, and courses across the rotator interval to the lesser tuberosity adjacent to the bicipital groove. The superior glenohumeral ligament is the primary static restraint to inferior translation of the adducted shoulder. The coracohumeral ligament is an extra-articular structure that arises from the base of the coracoid and passes between the

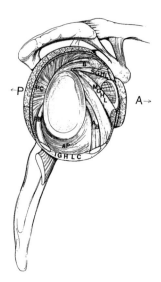

Fig. 1. Schematic drawing of the shoulder capsule showing the glenohumeral ligaments highlighting the inferior glenohumoral ligament complex (IGHLC). A, anterior; P, posterior; B, biceps tendon; AB, anterior band; AP, axillary pouch; PB, posterior band; PC, posterior capsule. (*From* O'Brien SJ, Neves MC, Arnoczky SP, et al. The anatomy and histology of the inferior glenohumeral ligament complex of the shoulder. Am J Sports Med 1990;18:449–56; with permission.)

supraspinatus and subscapularis, forming the roof of the rotator interval. It is composed of an anterior and posterior band that inserts onto the lesser and greater tuberosity, respectively. The coracohumeral ligament is a static restraint to anteroinferior translation in the adducted shoulder. The middle glenohumeral ligament has the most variable morphology of the ligaments; however, no distinct variation in its structure has been correlated with increased rates of instability. The middle glenohumeral ligament originates in the upper third of the anterior glenoid rim and labrum and courses obliquely across the subscapularis tendon to its humeral attachment on the lesser tuberosity. The middle glenohumeral ligament prevents anterior translation when the shoulder is externally rotated and in the middle range of abduction. The inferior glenohumeral ligament complex consists of an anterior and posterior band and the axillary pouch. It originates from the inferior labrum and inserts on to the humeral neck. Turkel and colleagues [12] demonstrated that the anterior band of the inferior glenohumeral ligament is the primary restraint to anterior glenohumeral translation with the arm in an abducted and externally rotated position. Anterior dislocation usually results from an indirect force with the arm in the abducted, externally rotated position. In this position, the anterior band of the inferior glenohumeral ligament is tensioned across the front of the glenoid (Fig. 2). In conjunction with the labrum, this normally prevents further anterior translation of the humeral head. With sufficient force during an anterior dislocation, however, the anterior band of the inferior glenohumeral ligament is detached and is referred to as a "Bankart lesion." This "essential" lesion is the pathoanatomic feature of anterior instability and its anatomic repair is the basis of any stabilization procedure.

A traumatic anterior shoulder dislocation typically results in posterolateral humeral head compression against the bony glenoid rim. This produces the classic Hill-Sachs lesion (Fig. 3), a chondral or osteochondral compression fracture. A large Hill-Sachs lesion may engage the anterior glenoid with humeral abduction and external rotation. Repeated episodes of an engaging Hill-Sachs lesion on the anterior glenoid can lead to anterior glenoid bone loss, which can worsen the instability. These lesions are considered pathognomonic for anterior instability and typically can be appreciated on plain radiographs.

Clinical evaluation

Multiple static and dynamic structures contribute to shoulder stability; proper evaluation including a thorough history, physical examination, and appropriate imaging studies is essential to identify injured structures and plan treatment. Shoulder instability is classified by the degree, frequency, etiology, and direction of instability. Patient history and physical examination should focus on accurately classifying the instability pattern. This article focuses on anterior glenohumeral dislocation and instability.

History

A careful history is essential to begin to classify the patient's instability. The cause of the instability may be readily apparent because the patient may describe a frank traumatic dislocation event, a history of repetitive microtrauma with overhead activity, or generalized laxity that may be familial. Patients are usually able clearly to describe the

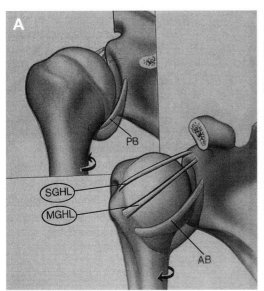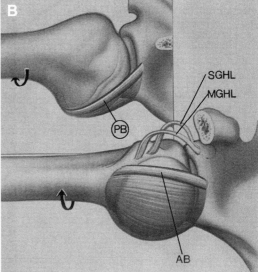

Fig. 2. The glenohumeral ligaments provide static restraint in different functional positions. (*A*) With the shoulder in adduction and external rotation, the superior glenohumeral ligament (SGHL) and the middle glenohumeral ligament (MGHL) are taut, whereas the anterior band (AB) and posterior band (PB) of the IGHLC are lax. (*B*) With the shoulder in abduction and external rotation, the AB of the IGHLC tightens and the SGHL and MGHL become lax. (*From* Warren RF, Craig EV, Altchek DW. The unstable shoulder. Philadelphia: Lippincott-Ravens; 1999. p. 65; with permission.)

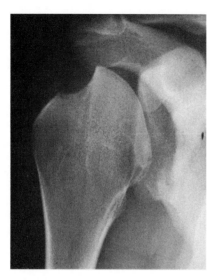

Fig. 3. Anteroposterior radiograph of a right shoulder demonstrating a Hill-Sachs lesion.

frequency and chronicity of instability episodes. Pain or instability with particular movements or positions may reveal the direction of instability. Patients with anterior instability report symptoms with the arm in an abducted and externally rotated position: the apprehension position. This is in contrast to posterior instability, which often occurs with the arm flexed, internally rotated, and adducted. Patients with inferior instability often have pain while carrying heavy objects; they may also experience traction paresthesias. Although anterior instability is by far more common than other directions, posterior instability and multidirectional instability may occur and should always be ruled out. Finally, it is important to inquire about symptoms at night. A patient who reports instability or a frank dislocation while sleeping most likely has severe instability and is more likely to fail conservative management compared with the patient who only experiences symptoms with activity.

Physical examination

Examination of the shoulder in a patient with instability begins with a thorough evaluation of the cervical spine for range of motion and any evidence of nerve root impingement. Next, one should carefully inspect the shoulder girdle and upper extremity, which may reveal obvious deformity. Anterior dislocations are characterized by prominence of the humeral head anterior, medial, and often inferior to the shoulder joint. A hollow region beneath the lateral deltoid can easily be palpated and the patient usually presents holding the arm in a position of adduction and internal rotation. In patients who do not have any obvious deformity, one proceeds with the examination. The authors routinely palpate the sternoclavicular joint, acromioclavicular joint, and biceps tendon to identify any areas of pain. Range of motion is assessed in varying degrees of shoulder adduction and typically in 90 degrees of abduction. The examiner should evaluate internal rotation, external rotation, abduction, and forward elevation in the scapular plane. Both limbs should be examined at the same time so that one can compare the injured with the noninjured side and the dominant with nondominant side. Motor strength is then tested and the extremity is examined for gross neurovascular deficits. The presence of rotator cuff pathology, especially in older patients, is then evaluated before proceeding toward specific maneuvers to diagnose instability.

Stability should be tested in the anterior, posterior, and inferior directions. These tests are always performed on both shoulders so that the results can be referenced to the unaffected side. With stability testing, it is important that the patient be as relaxed as possible. It is important to note that although these tests are used primarily to assess for instability, grinding, clicking, or pain can be common and may represent labral tears or chondral defects. Start by examining for inferior displacement with the patient seated and attempt to elicit a sulcus sign. This is performed by stabilizing the scapula with one hand and then applying longitudinal traction on the distal humerus with the other. This test is graded by measuring the size of the sulcus created from the inferior separation of the humeral head in relation to the acromion. A 1+ sulcus is equivalent to 1 cm of inferior translation. A 2+ sulcus is equivalent to 2 cm of displacement and may be seen in throwers or professional dancers. A 3+ sulcus or greater than 3 cm displacement is abnormal and associated with pathologic instability often in the form of multidirectional instability.

Provocative maneuvers include the apprehension test (performed supine) and the crank test (performed seated or upright). The patient is placed supine for the anterior apprehension test and the shoulder is positioned in maximum

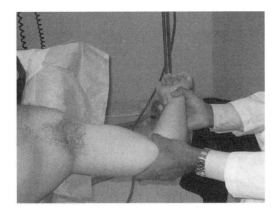

Fig. 4. Apprehension test for instability.

abduction and external rotation (Fig. 4). A positive test occurs when the patient exhibits guarding or discomfort and becomes "apprehensive" about the shoulder in this position. It should be noted that pain in this position is different from the feeling that the shoulder is going to come out of the joint. This distinction is important because this position may elicit pain in patients with internal impingement or other pathology. With the patient still supine, one can perform the relocation test for instability. With the shoulder still in full abduction and external rotation, a posteriorly directed force is applied, which causes the apprehension to disappear in patients with anterior instability (Fig. 5). The authors have found this test to lack specificity [13].

Perform the load and shift test to determine the degree of translation of the shoulder. This test can be performed in the seated or supine position and at various levels of glenohumeral abduction. The authors prefer to perform this test in the supine position (Fig. 6); with one hand, the examiner applies an axial load to the elbow to keep the humeral head centered on the glenoid. With the other hand, the examiner then applies an anterior and posteriorly directed force to assess how much translation of the humerus occurs on the glenoid. The test is performed with the arm at the side, at 45 degrees, and at 90 degrees. Persistent translation with increasing degrees of abduction may indicate compromise of the inferior glenohumeral ligament or capsulolabral structures. Grading the translation is based on comparing the injured shoulder with the opposite side and is as follows: 1+ is increased translation compared with the opposite side; 2+ is when the humeral head can be translated over the rim of the glenoid with spontaneous reduction; and 3+ is when the humeral head can be translated over the rim of the glenoid and stays there [14]. This classification applies to both anterior and posterior directions. The load and shift test has more clinical value in the operating room at the time of the examination under anesthesia because guarding during an office visit may limit the evaluation.

Imaging

Acute traumatic shoulder dislocations are evaluated with a trauma series that includes an anteroposterior, a transscapular (Y) lateral, and an axillary view. The axillary view is especially important to confirm reduction. In more chronic instability, additional views are useful to assess bony anatomy and identify characteristic

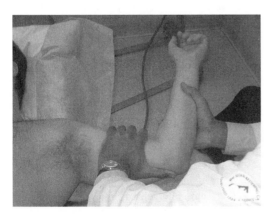

Fig. 5. Relocation test for instability.

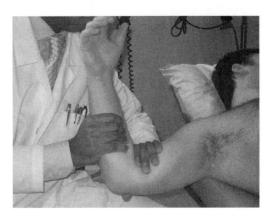

Fig. 6. The load and shift test for instability is a test for laxity or translation of the shoulder.

pathologic lesions. The West Point axillary view shows the anterior glenoid rim and may reveal bony Bankart lesions. The Stryker notch view shows the posterosuperior humeral head and can identify Hill-Sachs lesions. CT scans are obtained in selected patients with complex bony injuries and occasionally to evaluate the glenoid and humeral head version.

MRI has become the gold standard for evaluating the soft tissue injuries associated with anterior stability. With MRI, capsular and ligament detachments, labral lesions, rotator cuff tears, articular cartilage lesions, and osseous injury in the form of translational contusions can be identified with more accuracy than with radiographs or CT scan. Recently, the use of intra-articular gadolinium further to elucidate glenohumeral pathoanatomy has added an additional dimension to conventional MRI. Some authors have found magnetic resonance arthrography to be better than MRI without gadolinium enhancement for diagnosing capsulolabral injury [15,16]. At the authors' institution, noncontrast MRI has become the standard advanced imaging modality for diagnosing capsulolabral pathology in patients with anterior glenohumeral instability (Fig. 7). Although previous studies have reported that noncontrast MRI is not as accurate as magnetic resonance arthrography, the authors' experience has been that high-resolution noncontrast MRI can accurately diagnose capsulobral and bony injuries in patients with glenohumeral instability [17].

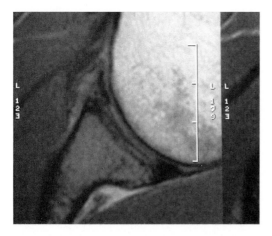

Fig. 7. Axial view of a noncontrast MRI demonstrating a Bankart lesion.

Treatment

Nonoperative management: acute shoulder dislocation

Acute dislocations should be reduced as quickly and atraumatically as possible. After a trauma series is obtained, closed reduction is performed with the patient relaxed with sedation or local anesthetics. When an athlete sustains an anterior dislocation that is evaluated on the field, it is most appropriate to attempt a reduction in a timely manner without necessarily obtaining prereduction radiographs. After reduction of the dislocation, management of an acute shoulder dislocation consists of a variable period of immobilization followed by rehabilitation focused on restoration of active motion and periscapular muscle strengthening. Traditionally, after closed reduction of a glenohumeral dislocation, patients were placed in a simple shoulder sling in internal rotation. Some recent reports, however, have suggested that immobilization in a position of humeral external rotation may result in a lower rate of recurrence compared with traditional immobilization in internal rotation [18,19]. Additionally, a recent MRI study demonstrated that immobilization of the arm in external rotation better approximates the Bankart lesion to the glenoid neck than does the conventional position of internal rotation [20]. In a randomized controlled trial, Itoi and colleagues [21] demonstrated that immobilization in external rotation after an initial shoulder dislocation reduced the risk of recurrence compared with that associated with the conventional method of immobilization in internal rotation. In contrast, a recent cadaveric study seems to refute the concept that external rotation should be more effective at approximating the labrum to the glenoid [22]. This concept needs to be evaluated further before adopting immobilization in external rotation as the standard of care.

After an acute anterior shoulder dislocation, the authors recommend immobilization in a sling for comfort for about 1 week, followed by range of motion exercises as tolerated with progression to strengthening exercises. During this rehabilitation process, an emphasis is placed on periscapular muscle strengthening. The improvement in periscapular and dynamic stabilizer (lower subscapulairs, pectoralis major, and latissimus dorsi) muscle strength and propioception may occasionally allow a patient to function with instability.

Orthotics that limit humeral abduction or external rotation can be used to allow an athlete to complete a season [23], although this should be considered carefully to weigh the potential for further damage.

Operative management: first-time shoulder dislocations

Numerous studies have demonstrated that conventional, nonoperative treatment of shoulder dislocations in young athletes has resulted in a high rate of recurrence. In patients under 30 years of age nonoperative management, which includes a period of immobilization followed by rehabilitation, has resulted in rates as high as 96% [1–5]. As a result, some researchers have investigated the role of arthroscopic treatment in first-time shoulder dislocations. Wheeler and colleagues [24] reported a 22% failure rate in West Point cadets after arthroscopic Bankart repair compared with a 92% failure rate for patients with nonoperative treatment. Arciero and colleagues [25] reported a 14% failure in the operatively treated group compared with an 80% failure rate in the nonoperative group. In two prospective, randomized studies of young, first-time dislocators, Kirkley and colleagues [26] and Bottoni and colleagues [27] reported significantly lower recurrence rates following arthroscopic Bankart repair when compared with nonoperative treatment. Additionally, patients treated surgically demonstrated a superior outcome compared with the nonoperative group using a quality-of-life assessment.

From these studies, it seems that operative treatment for primary dislocations in a young population may reduce recurrence, improve outcome, and avoid the frequent necessity of open reconstructive procedures in patients who suffer from recurrent instability. Although the rate of recurrence is high in the young active population, it is not 100%. A small number of patients may be treated surgically unnecessarily. The authors recommend arthroscopic stabilization after primary anterior shoulder dislocation in young athletic patients who are unwilling to modify their activities because they believe that the risks incurred by nonoperative treatment (eg, high rate of recurrence, disability following each instability episode, and the potential for more significant injury and associated pathology including articular cartilage damage) outweigh those incurred by surgery.

Operative management: recurrent instability

The goals for treatment of shoulder instability (to restore the anatomy) are identical whether the procedure is arthroscopic or open: to repair the avulsion of the anteroinferior capsulolabral complex anatomically and to address capsular injury that can occur at the time of the instability episode. All patients should be examined in the operating room, under anesthesia, before surgery to assess the glenohumeral stability. This allows for a more accurate assessment of instability because the patients have complete muscular paralysis and are not guarded. After an examination under anesthesia, a diagnostic shoulder arthroscopy should be performed to assess the intra-articular anatomy, confirm the presence of a Bankart lesion, and contrast intraoperative findings with preoperative imaging. The goal of the procedure is to restore the anatomy and address associated pathology. The authors' approach has been primarily arthroscopic reconstructions in recent years. If there are large bone deficiencies on either the humeral or glenoid side, arthrotomy may be necessary, although these are uncommon.

Arthroscopic stabilization

The authors perform shoulder arthroscopy with the patient in the beach chair position. The patient is anesthetized under intrascalene or supraclavicular block with sedation. After a complete examination under anesthesia is performed, a 30-degree arthroscope is introduced into the glenohumeral joint by the posterior portal. A standard anterior portal is established in the rotator interval and a complete diagnostic arthroscopy is performed. A probe is used to confirm the presence of a Bankart lesion and the extent of any other concomitant pathology is assessed (Fig. 8). At this time, a decision is made on whether to proceed with an arthroscopic repair or convert to an open procedure. This decision is based on the presence of osseous insufficiency and the quality of the tissue for repair. If the decision is made to proceed with an arthroscopic repair, a second anteroinferior portal is established just superior to the subscapularis tendon. This portal, the working portal, is confirmed first by spinal needle localization and should allow direct access to the Bankart lesion. An arthroscopic elevator is used to release the labrum from the glenoid in preparation for the repair (Fig. 9). Next, any unstable flaps of labrum are debrided to a stable

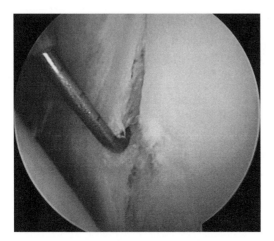

Fig. 8. Arthroscopic picture with probe confirming a Bankart lesion.

rim and an arthroscopic shaver or burr is used to prepare the anteroinferior glenoid to a rim of bleeding bone. After the bed of the Bankart lesion has been adequately prepared, a nonmetallic suture anchor is then inserted by the working portal into the anterior-inferior aspect of the glenoid off the face. The anchors are placed beginning at the inferior aspect of the glenoid first. The medial limb from the suture anchor is retrieved into the anterior portal. A monofilament suture is passed through the capsule and labrum using an angled suture-passing instrument. The end of the passing

suture, which is in the defect, is then retrieved through the anterior portal. The two sutures are tied outside the shoulder and the opposite limb of the PDS suture is pulled, which shuttles the medial limb of the suture anchor through the capsulolabral tissue. The suture anchor limbs are then tied using an arthroscopic sliding knot thereby securing the tissue to the bone (Fig. 10). The labrum is probed for stability and security of fixation and this process is repeated as necessary.

Open stabilization

The beach chair position for the diagnostic arthroscopy allows for easy conversion to the open procedure when indicated. The operative extremity can be supported on a padded Mayo stand or a commercially available arm holder. The decision to convert to open stabilization is based on many factors, including the presence of large engaging osseous lesions, which may need to be addressed; excessive capsular redundancy as encountered with multidirectional instability; or poor quality of capsular tissue, which may necessitate the use of autograft or allograft supplementation. An incision is made in the axilla for improved cosmesis (Fig. 11), and through a deltopectoral approach the cephalic vein is identified and retracted laterally. A self-retaining retractor is placed laterally underneath the deltoid and medially underneath the pectoralis major. In select cases the superior portion of the pectoralis major may be incised for exposure and repaired later. The clavipectoral fascia is then incised and the strap muscles are carefully retracted medially.

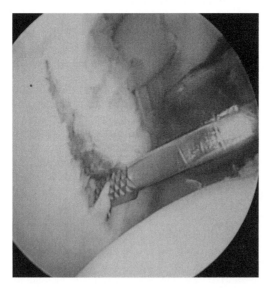

Fig. 9. An arthroscopic elevator is used to release the labrum from the glenoid in preparation for the repair.

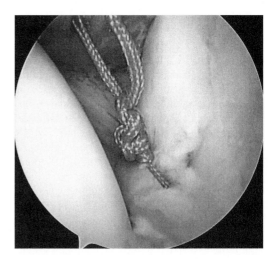

Fig. 10. Arthroscopic image of one suture anchor that has been tied after capsular placation.

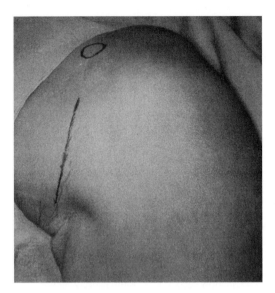

Fig. 11. For open stabilizations, an incision in the axilla is used for improved cosmesis.

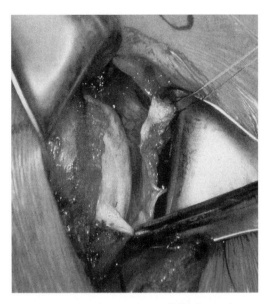

Fig. 12. The capsule must be carefully dissected away from the subscapularis so that a capular shift can be performed after the Bankart repair to eliminate redundancy.

Care must be taken to avoid injury to the musculocutaneous nerve. The anterior humeral circumflex vessels are cauterized to maintain hemostasis and prepare the approach through the subscapularis tendon. The approach through the subscapularis may be performed by releasing the tendon approximately 1 cm from the insertion on the lesser tuberosity or by performing a split through the muscle as described by Jobe and coworkers [28], although most cases that are indicated for this latter approach are now repaired arthroscopically. With the arm in adduction and slight external rotation, the subscapularis tendon is longitudinally sectioned and carefully separated from the underlying capsule.

The capsular approach may be performed laterally [29], medially [30], or in the midline [31]. The authors prefer the humeral-based capsular approach from the lateral side. This affords a greater ability to shift the capsule in cases of multidirectional instability. The medial-based approach provides direct access to the Bankart lesion but may not provide the capacity to shift as much capsule. The midline approach places the axillary nerve at greater risk because the capsular incision is performed in proximity to the nerve's location.

A longitudinal capsulotomy is made approximately 5 mm medial to the humeral capsular insertion (Fig. 12). A horizontal capsular incision can then be made perpendicular to the capsulotomy in cases in which an inferior capsular shift is also being performed. When there is less capsular redundancy, the horizontal split in the capsule is not necessary. A humeral head retractor is then levered on the posterior edge of the glenoid to displace the humeral head posteriorly and laterally to maintain optimal visualization and exposure in preparation of the Bankart lesion. Anatomic labral repair is then performed using suture anchors. Typically three anchors are used to repair the Bankart lesion. Following repair, a capsular shift is used to eliminate capsular redundancy while the humeral head is maintained in at least 45 degrees of abduction and 45 degrees of external rotation. The capsule is then repaired using either the inferior capsular shift technique by advancing the inferior leaflet superiorly along the lateral capsular margin and then reinforcing the repair with the overlapping superior leaflet, or by repairing the capsule in its entirety to the humeral side with a slight superior shift in cases with less capsular volume. An adequate capsular shift is accomplished when the capsular redundancy is eliminated through superior advancement of the inferior capsular shift. Anatomic repair of the subscapularis is then performed in an end-to-end fashion with the previously placed sutures.

Postoperative rehabilitation

Following anterior stabilization with either an arthroscopic or an open procedure, the authors immobilize patients in a simple shoulder immobilizer for 4 weeks. During this time period, pendulum exercises and active range of motion of the elbow are permitted. At 4 weeks, patients progress to supine forward elevation in the scapular plane to 140 degrees and external rotation is limited to 45 degrees. Active and passive range of motion of the elbow and wrist are continued and the sling is discontinued at 4 to 6 weeks. After 6 weeks, forward elevation and external rotation are progressed as tolerated and strengthening exercises that emphasize the posterior rotator cuff, latissimus, and periscapular muscles are begun. All strength exercises are performed below the horizontal plane. At 12 weeks, aggressive scapular stabilization and eccentric strengthening are begun and from 4 to 6 months patients proceed to sports-specific strengthening and proprioception with a gradual return to sporting activities after 6 months depending on return of function and strength. Slight modifications by the therapist is allowed based on each individual's progress.

Results

The open Bankart repair is historically the gold standard for stabilization procedures and the benchmark against which all arthroscopic techniques are measured. The failure rates after open shoulder stabilization for recurrent anterior instability have been reported to be 3% to 9% [32]. Rowe and colleagues [33] in 1978 reported a 3% failure rate in 143 shoulders after open stabilization. This paper, like most studies, defined failure as a second dislocation and lacked patient-focused outcomes and objective functional criteria. Over time, the criteria for failure have broadened to include functional criteria, such as the ability to return to preinjury activity level. Bigliani and colleagues [34] in 1994 reported only 67% of 63 throwing athletes were able to return to their preinjury levels of competition after an open Bankart repair. Additionally, postoperative loss of motion after shoulder stabilization, for example, needs to be taken into account after shoulder stabilization because it is possible that the low rate of secondary dislocation after open procedure may be a result of limited glenohumeral motion, which can be more disabling than recurrent instability. Perhaps the failure rate of many of the traditional studies with open procedures would be higher if "failure" was broadened to include more subjective and objective patient outcome measures.

Many studies have attempted to assess the results of arthroscopic stabilization using a variety of techniques [24–27,35–37]. Nearly all of them demonstrated that arthroscopic stabilization resulted in a higher rate of recurrent instability when compared with traditional open techniques. Again, failure in almost all these studies was determined solely by recurrent instability. Additionally, all of these studies were conducted during the early stages of arthroscopic stabilization. As the experience and equipment in shoulder arthroscopy has improved, several authors have tried directly to compare arthroscopic and open stabilization procedures. Kim and colleagues [38] in a retrospective evaluation of open and arthroscopic stabilization reported excellent results in almost 90% of all patients in both groups. Currently, there are three studies that have prospectively compared arthroscopic and open repairs. First, Cole and colleagues [39] compared arthroscopic and open repairs and found comparable results at a mean follow-up of more than 52 months. Fabbriciani and colleagues [40] in a prospective evaluation of open and arthroscopic repairs in 60 patients reported no recurrent instability in patients from either group. Lastly, Bottoni and colleagues [41] recently reported on a consecutive series of 64 patients who were prospectively randomized to either arthroscopic or open stabilization. They concluded that clinical outcomes were comparable; however, the mean loss of motion was greater in the open shoulders, although this difference was not statistically significant.

These results suggest that both open and arthroscopic Bankart repairs are safe and reliable in returning most patients with recurrent instability to full preinjury activity levels. Given that both techniques work, it has been the authors' preference to use arthroscopic repair for the treatment of recurrent anterior shoulder instability.

Summary

Anterior shoulder dislocation is a common problem encountered by the orthopedic surgeon. The age of the patient at the time of the first dislocation is inversely related to the recurrence rate and clearly influences treatment recommendations. The data suggest that younger athletic patients who are unwilling to modify their activities should receive stabilization after their initial dislocation to avoid recurrent instability. Except in the young athlete, nonoperative management should be the initial course of treatment followed by a supervised rehabilitation program; however, when indicated, operative stabilization can predictably allow patients to return to preinjury function in a high percentage of patients. Patients who suffer from instability should undergo a thorough preoperative work-up to identify the cause of the instability and any concomitant shoulder pathology. Whether an open or arthroscopic technique is chosen, careful attention to operative principles is imperative for a successful outcome. Arthroscopic stabilization can be as successful as the traditional open procedure with the added benefit of reduced operative time, better cosmesis, and improved range of motion. It is a technically demanding procedure, however, and should only be performed by an experienced arthroscopist.

References

[1] Henry JH, Genung JA. Natural history of glenohumeral dislocation: revisited. Am J Sports Med 1982;10:135–7.

[2] Hovelius L. Anterior shoulder dislocation of the shoulder in teen-agers and young adults: five-year prognosis. J Bone Joint Surg Am 1987;69A:393–9.

[3] Hovelius L. Shoulder dislocation in Swedish ice hockey players. Am J Sports Med 1978;6:373–7.

[4] Hovelius L, Augustini BG, Fredin H, et al. Primary anterior dislocation of the shoulder in young patients: a ten-year prospective study. J Bone Joint Surg 1996;78A:1677–84.

[5] Hovelius L, Eriksson K, Fredin H, et al. Recurrences after initial dislocation of the shoulder: results of a prospective study of treatment. J Bone Joint Surg 1983;65A:343–9.

[6] Rowe CR, Sakellarides HT. Factors related to recurrences of anterior dislocations of the shoulder. Clin Orthop 1961;20:40–8.

[7] Simonet WT, Cofield RH. Prognosis in anterior shoulder dislocation. Am J Sports Med 1984;12:19–24.

[8] Howell SM, Galinat BJ, Renzi AJ, et al. Normal and abnormal mechanics of the glenohumeral joint in the horizontal motion plane. J Bone Joint Surg 1988;70A:227–32.

[9] Poppen NK, Walker PS. Normal and abnormal motion of the shoulder. J Bone Joint Surg 1976;58A:195–201.

[10] Cordasco FA, Wolfe IN, Wooten ME, et al. An electromyographic analysis of the shoulder during a medicine ball rehabilitation program. Am J Sports Med 1996;24(3):386–92.

[11] Howell SM, Galinat BJ. The glenoid-labral socket. Clin Orthop Relat Res 1989;243:122–5.

[12] Turkel SJ, Panio MW, Marshall JL, et al. Stabilizing mechanisms preventing anterior dislocation of the glenohumeral joint. J Bone Joint Surg 1981;63:1208–17.

[13] Speer KP, Hannafin JA, Altchek DW, et al. An evaluation of the shoulder relocation test. Am J Sports Med 1994;22(2):177–83.

[14] Altchek DW, Dines DM. Shoulder injuries in the throwing athlete. J Am Acad Orthop Surg 1995;3:159–65.

[15] Chandnani VP, Gagliardi JA, Murnane TG, et al. Glenohumeral ligaments and shoulder capsular mechanisms: evaluation with MR arthrography. Radiology 1995;196:27–32.

[16] Chandnani VP, Yeager TD, DeBerardino T, et al. Glenoid labral tears: prospective evaluation with MRI imaging, MR arthrography, and CT arthrography. Am J Roentgenol 1993;161:1229–35.

[17] Gusmer PB, Potter HG, Schatz JA, et al. Labral injuries: accuracy of detection with unenhanced MR imaging of the shoulder. Radiology 1996;200(2):519–24.

[18] Itoi E, Hatakeyama Y, Kido T, et al. A new method of immobilization after traumatic anterior dislocation of the shoulder: a preliminary study. J Shoulder Elbow Surg 2003;12:413–5.

[19] Seybold D, Gekyle C, Fehmer T. Immobilization in external rotation after primary shoulder dislocation. Chirurg 2006;77(9):821–6.

[20] Itoi E, Sashi R, Minagawa H, et al. Position of immobilization after dislocation of the glenohumeral joint: a study with use of magnetic resonance imaging. J Bone Joint Surg 2001;83A:661–7.

[21] Itoi E, Hatakeyama Y, Sato T, et al. Immobilization in external rotation after shoulder dislocation reduces the risk of recurrence: a randomized controlled trial. J Bone Joint Surg 2007;89(10):2124–31.

[22] Limpisvasti O, Yang BY, Hosseinzadeh P, et al. The Effect of glenohumeral position on the shoulder following traumatic anterior dislocation. Am J Sports Med 2008;36(4):775–80.

[23] Buss DD, Lynch GP, Meyer CP, et al. Nonoperative management for in-season athletes with anterior shoulder instability. Am J Sports Med 2004;32(6):1430–3.

[24] Wheeler JH, Ryan JB, Arciero RA, et al. Arthroscopic versus nonoperative treatment of acute shoulder dislocations in young athletes. Arthroscopy 1989;5:213–7.

[25] Arciero RA, Wheeler JH, Ryan JB, et al. Arthroscopic Bankart repair versus nonoperative treatment for acute, initial anterior shoulder dislocations. Am J Sports Med 1994;22:589–94.

[26] Kirkley A, Griffin S, Richards C, et al. Prospective randomized clinical trial comparing the effectiveness of immediate arthroscopic stabilization versus immobilization and rehabilitation in first traumatic anterior dislocations of the shoulder. Arthroscopy 1999;15:507–14.

[27] Bottoni CR, Wilckens JH, DeBerardino TM, et al. A prospective, randomized, evaluation of arthroscopic stabilization versus nonoperative treatment of acute, first-time shoulder dislocations. Am J Sports Med 2002;30(4):576–80.

[28] Jobe FW, Giangarra CE, Kvitne RS, et al. Anterior capsulolabral reconstruction of the shoulder in athletes in overhand sports. Am J Sports Med 1991; 19(5):428–34.

[29] Neer CS II, Foster CR. Inferior capsular shift for involuntary inferior and multidirectional instability of the shoulder: a preliminary report. J Bone Joint Surg 1980;62(6):897–908.

[30] Altchek DW, Warren RF, Skyhar MJ, et al. T-plasty modification of the Bankart procedure for multidirectional instability of the anterior and inferior types. J Bone Joint Surg 1991;73(1): 105–12.

[31] Wirth MA, Blatter G, Rockwood CA Jr. The capsular imbrication procedure for recurrent anterior instability of the shoulder. J Bone Joint Surg 1996; 78(2):246–59.

[32] Bigliani LU. Recurrent anterior instability: open surgical repair. In: Bigliani LU, editor. The unstable shoulder. Rosemont (IL): American Academy of Orthopaedic Surgeons; 1996. p. 59–67.

[33] Rowe CR, Patel D, Southmayd WW. The Bankart procedure: a long-term end-result study. J Bone Joint Surg 1978;60:1–16.

[34] Bigliani LU, Kurzweil PR, Schwartzbach CC, et al. Inferior capsular shift procedure for anterior-inferior shoulder instability in athletes. Am J Sports Med 1994;22:578–84.

[35] Arciero RA, Taylor DC. Primary anterior dislocation of the shoulder in young patients: a ten-year prospective study. J Bone Joint Surg Am 1998;80:299–300.

[36] Baker CL, Uribe JW, Whitman C. Arthroscopic evaluation of acute initial anterior shoulder dislocations. Am J Sports Med 1990;18:25–8.

[37] DeBerardino TM, Arciero RA, Taylor DC. Arthroscopic stabilization of acute initial anterior shoulder dislocation: the West Point experience. J South Orthop Assoc 1996;5:263–71.

[38] Kim SH, Ha KI, Kim SH. Bankart repair in traumatic anterior shoulder instability: open versus arthroscopic technique. Arthroscopy 2002;18:755–63.

[39] Cole BJ, L'Insalata J, Irrgang J, et al. Comparison of arthroscopic and open anterior shoulder stabilization: a two-to-six year follow-up study. J Bone Joint Surg Am 2000;82:1108–14.

[40] Fabbriciani C, Milano G, Demontis A, et al. Arthroscopic versus open treatment of Bankart lesion of the shoulder: a prospective randomized study. Arthroscopy 2004;20:456–62.

[41] Bottoni CR, Smith EL, Berkowitz MJ, et al. Arthroscopic versus open shoulder stabilization for recurrent anterior instability. Am J Sports Med 2005; 34(11):1730–7.

ELSEVIER
SAUNDERS

Orthop Clin N Am 39 (2008) 519–533

ORTHOPEDIC
CLINICS
OF NORTH AMERICA

Traumatic Posterior Glenohumeral Dislocation: Classification, Pathoanatomy, Diagnosis, and Treatment

Marc S. Kowalsky, MD, William N. Levine, MD*

Department of Orthopaedic Surgery, Center for Shoulder, Elbow, and Sports Medicine, Columbia University Medical Center, 622 W. 168th Street, PH-1117, New York, NY 10032, USA

Posterior glenohumeral dislocations represent approximately 2% to 5% of all traumatic shoulder dislocations [1–4]. A precise determination of the incidence remains difficult because of the frequency with which posterior dislocations go undetected. Proposed explanations for the delay in diagnosis include failure of the evaluating physician to include the condition in the differential diagnosis, suboptimal radiographic evaluation and interpretation, and coincidental injuries such as fractures that can confound the patient's presentation [5].

More than 5 decades ago, McLaughlin [3] recognized these pitfalls in the diagnosis of posterior glenohumeral dislocation when he said, "clinical and roentgenographic evidence of this lesion is always present, but usually escapes notice unless deduced." The delay in diagnosis and subsequent treatment of this injury often jeopardizes the potential effectiveness of any orthopedic intervention. Thus, the delay in diagnosis, the complexity of these injuries, and their rarity contribute to the significant morbidity associated with posterior glenohumeral dislocations.

It is imperative that orthopedic surgeons develop a complete understanding of the nature of this injury and its treatment so that patients who present with this condition can be diagnosed and treated effectively. This article provides a detailed discussion of the classification, pathoanatomy, diagnosis, and treatment of traumatic posterior glenohumeral dislocation.

Classification

In part because of the rarity of posterior glenohumeral dislocation, most of the available literature treating this condition consists of level IV or level V evidence. Therefore, although countless classification systems have been proposed, none has emerged as the definitive instrument with which to approach this condition in the context of academic research or clinical practice. May [6] proposed a straightforward distinction among habitual, traumatic, and obstetric posterior dislocation or subluxation, but this simple classification did not address the true complexity of this condition and therefore has been abandoned in favor of more complex proposals.

In his proposed classification system, Detenbeck [1] included chronicity as a factor to consider in the natural history and management of posterior glenohumeral dislocation. He distinguished among acute, chronic, and recurrent posterior instability and further subdivided recurrent instability into traumatic and atraumatic variants. Hawkins and Bell [7] expanded this classification system further. They distinguished between acute posterior dislocations that are associated with an impression defect and those that are not. Further, they classified recurrent subluxation as a form of chronic dislocation and distinguished this variant from a locked, or missed, chronic dislocation associated with an impression defect. Moreover,

---

* Corresponding author.

E-mail address: wnl1@columbia.edu (W.N. Levine).

they distinguished voluntary and involuntary recurrent subluxation.

Heller and colleagues [8] have offered perhaps the most comprehensive classification of posterior glenohumeral dislocations. They include a discussion of an anatomic system of classification that distinguishes among subacromial, subglenoid, and subspinous posterior dislocation, but they concede that a strictly anatomic description offers very little assistance in developing a treatment strategy for this condition [9,10]. As the preferred alternative, they offer a definitive system of classification based on the underlying cause. They include all clinically relevant parameters in their classification: traumatic versus atraumatic, acute versus persistent, recurrent (posttraumatic versus atraumatic), and voluntary (posttraumatic versus atraumatic). This classification system was based on a review of 300 publications of 750 cases and thus represents the most comprehensive, widely applicable system offered to date.

Any classification system of posterior glenohumeral dislocation must include a careful discussion of the missed, locked, or persistent variety of dislocation. Because each of these terms is used with varying frequency and meanings, it is important to define them clearly. Hawkins and colleagues [11,12] and Robinson and Aderinto [5] have made perhaps the greatest contributions to the discussion and classification of persistent glenohumeral dislocation. They consider a dislocation acute if it occurred within 6 weeks and chronic if it has been present for more than 6 months. They also distinguished among persistent dislocations with impression defects of varying size. They recognize that the size of this impression defect determines the optimal treatment strategy and thus defined the following categories: less than 20%, between 20% to 45%, and greater than 45% to 50%. This detailed classification of persistent posterior glenohumeral dislocation has provided valuable insight into the natural history and orthopedic management of this injury.

Robinson and colleagues [5,13] also have highlighted a significant aspect of posterior glenohumeral dislocation that had been overlooked in previous classification proposals. Because proximal and diaphyseal humerus fractures commonly are associated with posterior dislocation, one must distinguish between simple and complex dislocations. Robinson and colleagues [14] distinguished among the three most common types of complex dislocation and relied upon Neer's [15] original classification of proximal humerus fractures in their discussion. They include two-part fractures of the lesser tuberosity, two-part fractures of the anatomic neck, and three-part and four-part fractures of the proximal humerus.

Epidemiology

As noted earlier, posterior dislocation accounts for approximately 2% to 5% of all glenohumeral dislocations. The most recent review performed by Robinson and Aderinto [5] indicates that this number is closer to 3%. An accurate assessment of the incidence is challenging, however, because of the frequency with which this diagnosis is overlooked. In fact, the literature estimates that the diagnosis of posterior glenohumeral dislocation is missed in approximately 60% to 79% of cases [2]. One proposed explanation for missed diagnosis is that concomitant proximal humerus fracture can confound the patient's clinical presentation.

In fact, the incidence of complex posterior fracture-dislocation has been calculated to be 0.6 per 100,000 population per year [13]. Neer [14,15] estimated that this complex injury accounts for approximately 0.9% of all fractures and dislocations about the shoulder. Others have estimated that posterior fracture-dislocations involving the surgical neck account up to 50% of all posterior glenohumeral dislocations [16]. Most of these complex posterior glenohumeral fracture-dislocations include fracture of the tuberosities or the anatomic neck, alone or in combination [17–22]. The anatomic neck fracture represents propagation of the characteristic impression defect, or reverse Hill-Sachs defect, along the anterior aspect of the humeral articular surface. Although most complex injuries involve fracture of the proximal humerus, other associated fracture patterns have been described, including fracture of the acromion, the coracoid, or the humeral shaft [23,24]. An open posterior glenohumeral fracture-dislocation has been reported, resulting from high-energy trauma in a motor vehicle accident and associated with a brachial plexopathy [25]. Approximately 15% of all posterior glenohumeral dislocations are bilateral [26–34].

Unlike anterior dislocation, posterior glenohumeral dislocation associated with neurologic or vascular compromise is unusual [10]. With increasing severity of injury to the glenohumeral joint, however, the likelihood of neurologic compromise likewise increases. Reports of neurologic injury most often occur together with profound injury to the capsulolabral complex, rotator cuff, and the long head of the biceps tendon. The nerve most often affected is the axillary nerve, although injury to the suprascapular nerve can occur also [25,35].

Traumatic posterior glenohumeral dislocation may occur from an axial force applied to the upper extremity in the vulnerable position of adduction, internal rotation, and forward elevation [36]. Posterior dislocation, however, more commonly results from seizure activity during which contraction of the strong internal rotators of the glenohumeral joint overcomes the static and dynamic posterior stabilizers (Fig. 1). Classically, this mechanism occurs during a convulsive seizure in a patient who suffers from a seizure disorder [33,37]. Posterior dislocation secondary to seizure also may result from metabolic abnormalities such as hypoglycemia or hypocalcaemia [38,39]. Further, this injury pattern has been reported in patients who have experienced seizures secondary to alcohol withdrawal [5]. Intense muscle contraction secondary to electric shock or electroconvulsive shock therapy also has been reported to cause posterior glenohumeral dislocation [31,40]. Although anterior glenohumeral dislocation remains the most common direction of dislocation in all cohorts, regardless of mechanism, posterior dislocation in the absence of trauma most likely results from seizure or electric shock. Therefore, in patients presenting with posterior dislocation without known trauma, the orthopedic surgeon should maintain a strong suspicion for an underlying cause such as seizure disorder, metabolic disarray, or alcohol or drug withdrawal.

Pathoanatomy

A true understanding of the complexity of posterior dislocation requires a discussion of the normal functional anatomy of the glenohumeral joint. Static and dynamic structures confer posterior stability to the glenohumeral joint. Static stabilizers include the osseous anatomy of the shoulder. Although both the glenoid and humeral head are physiologically retroverted relative to the scapular and epicondylar axes (4°–7° and 30°–40°, respectively), the scapula is protracted on the chest wall 45°, which thus converts the glenoid to a partial posterior buttress to dislocation [7]. The glenoid, however, represents only approximately 25% to 30% of the articular surface the humeral head and thus has a limited ability to confer substantial stability.

The labrum overcomes this limitation to a certain extent by increasing the depth of the glenoid by approximately 50% [41]. In addition, the posterior capsule, together with the posterior band of the inferior glenohumeral ligament, provides static stability to the glenohumeral joint. Ovesen and Sojbjerg [42] found that all 10 cadaveric specimens subjected to posterior dislocation demonstrated rupture of the posterior capsule adjacent to the labrum. Weber and Caspari [43] confirmed these findings in a biomechanical study of nine cadaveric shoulders subjected to a posterior force in the vulnerable position. All shoulders demonstrated a lesion of the posterior capsule, six demonstrated an associated labral injury, and two demonstrated a glenoid rim fracture. The complement to an anterior labrum periosteal sleeve avulsion lesion, a posterior labrocapsular periosteal sleeve avulsion, has been associated with a locked posterior dislocation, confirming the importance of the posterior capsulolabral complex in posterior glenohumeral stability [44]. These biomechanical studies confirm that most of these lesions occur at the capsulolabral attachment on the glenoid, although a minority did occur at its attachment on the humerus.

Schwartz and colleagues [45] also performed cadaveric biomechanical studies to elucidate the role of the glenohumeral capsule and ligaments in posterior stability. Although incising the posterosuperior capsule alone did not lead to posterior

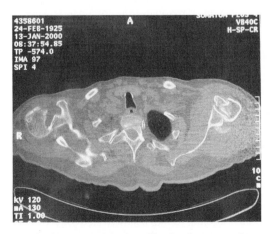

Fig. 1. A 52-year-old man suffered a first-ever seizure caused by a primary brain tumor that was diagnosed following the seizure and shoulder injury.

instability, propagation of the lesion to the entire posterior capsule did lead to posterior subluxation but not to frank dislocation. Posterior dislocation occurred only when the anterosuperior capsule, including the superior glenohumeral ligament, was incised also. Further, when the upper extremity is placed in the vulnerable position of flexion, adduction, and internal rotation, the anterior capsular structures became tense "like a cord." The authors concluded that the anterior structures served as a checkrein to posterior dislocation by tethering the humeral head in position. These investigators also were able to cause posterior instability by incising the entire inferior capsule, including the inferior glenohumeral ligament. As a result of these cadaveric experiments, the authors postulate that the static stabilizers of the glenohumeral joint should be conceptualized as a circular structure, in which attenuation of the anterior structures represents a critical component of the injury pattern allowing for posterior dislocation.

Dynamic structures that confer stability to the glenohumeral joint include the muscles of the shoulder girdle as well as the rotator cuff. In addition to injury to the posterior capsule, Ovesen and Sojbjerg [42] in their biomechanical study found a concomitant tear of the tendons of teres minor and infraspinatus. Hottya and colleagues [46] confirmed this finding in an imaging study of patients who had sustained posterior glenohumeral dislocation. All patients in the study demonstrated MRI evidence of injury to the teres minor, and half of the patients had a full-thickness rupture of this tendon. Injury to the posterosuperior rotator cuff also has been reported in association with posterior glenohumeral dislocation, although this pattern of injury is far more rare [47,48].

In addition to the characteristic posterior capsulolabral lesion, posterior glenohumeral dislocation creates a pathognomonic lesion in the humeral head. McLaughlin [3] described a distinctive vertical defect in the anterior aspect of the humeral head resulting from engagement of the posterior rim of the glenoid (Fig. 2). This defect results from direct traumatic impact, followed by resorption of subchondral bone of the proximal humeral articular surface. Consequently, the longer the glenohumeral joint remains dislocated, the longer the humeral head is subjected to this deforming force. The impression defect enlarges subsequently.

The significance of the humeral head impression defect is threefold. First, it serves as

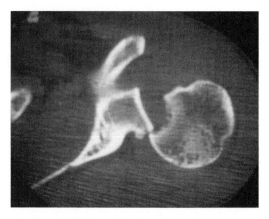

Fig. 2. Axial CT demonstrating characteristic anteromedial humeral head defect in a 32-year-old man after posterior dislocation.

a propagation point, rendering the proximal humerus susceptible to fracture of the anatomic neck, either at the time of injury or with subsequent iatrogenic displacement during a reduction maneuver. Second, the deformity of the humeral head articular surface resulting from this impression defect makes the glenohumeral joint susceptible to secondary osteoarthritis. Third, the size of the impression defect determines the stable arc of curvature of the glenohumeral articulation [16]. As the defect enlarges, it is exposed to the posterior glenoid rim at an earlier point in the glenohumeral arc of motion, rendering the glenohumeral joint susceptible to redislocation. Thus, a direct correlation exists between the defect size and joint stability. In turn, a determination of the defect size aids the orthopedic surgeon in developing the optimal treatment strategy for posterior glenohumeral dislocations.

Diagnosis

Although orthopedic surgeons rely heavily on diagnostic imaging in approaching patients who have musculoskeletal disease, clinical acumen together with a high index of suspicion are sufficient to diagnose posterior glenohumeral dislocation successfully. In fact, one of the earliest large series of such patients provided by Malgaigne [49] in 1855 relied on the history and physical examination alone. Mere inspection of the patient reveals certain characteristic traits of posterior dislocation. The patient presents with a prominent coracoid, an anterior glenohumeral void caused by the posterior position of the humeral head, and a squared-off anterolateral acromion and overlying soft tissue [2,3,11]. In more subtle cases of posterior instability, a skin dimple, which represents a tether of the postero-medial deltoid, may be found inferior and medial to the posterolateral edge of the acromion [50].

Examination of the patient's shoulder range of motion should suggest strongly the presence of the lesion. The injured extremity is held in internal rotation (Fig. 3). The patient also demonstrates marked limitations with respect to passive external rotation and abduction, because the humeral head remains impacted against the posterior glenoid rim. Because most physicians have an insufficient index of suspicion for this often-overlooked condition, this marked limitation of both active and passive range of motion often leads to the incorrect diagnosis of frozen shoulder, with resultant devastating consequences of delayed treatment of the dislocation. Hill and McLaughlin [51] reported a series of patients who had posterior glenohumeral dislocation and who were misdiagnosed as having frozen shoulder, or periarthritis. For these patients the delay in appropriate intervention averaged approximately 8 months and of course adversely affected the success of treatment. This morbidity always is avoidable by correct diagnosis based on sound clinical evaluation, together with an appropriate radiographic examination.

Inadequate roentgenographic evaluation represents perhaps the greatest barrier to the successful diagnosis of posterior glenohumeral dislocation. One can recognize most lesions about

the shoulder with anteroposterior and scapular lateral orthogonal views, but the untrained eye may miss subtle indices of posterior dislocation. Subtle signs of posterior dislocation have been described even though the gross glenohumeral relationships may remain well preserved. The humeral head is fixed in internal rotation (Fig. 4). Further, although a traditional antero-posterior view of the shoulder in the thoracic plane demonstrates slight overlap of the glenoid and humeral head, this half-moon crescentic overlap is absent in the case of posterior dislocation (Fig. 5) [36]. One also must examine a radiographic landmark referred to as "Moloney's line" (Fig. 6) [9]. This line runs along the inferior aspect of the glenoid rim and continues along the inferomedial aspect of the humeral head and neck. Analogous to Shenton's line in the evaluation of developmental dysplasia of the hip, Moloney's line is disrupted in posterior glenohumeral dislocation.

A complete radiographic evaluation of the shoulder in the context of possible posterior glenohumeral dislocation must include the trauma series described by Neer [14]: an anteroposterior view in the scapular plane, a scapular lateral view, and an axillary view. Hawkins [11] has stated that the axillary view alone is sufficient to confirm the diagnosis of posterior dislocation. The axillary view allows the evaluation of the glenoid and any glenoid rim fracture that may exist, as well as the estimation of the size of the impression defect and the amount of remaining

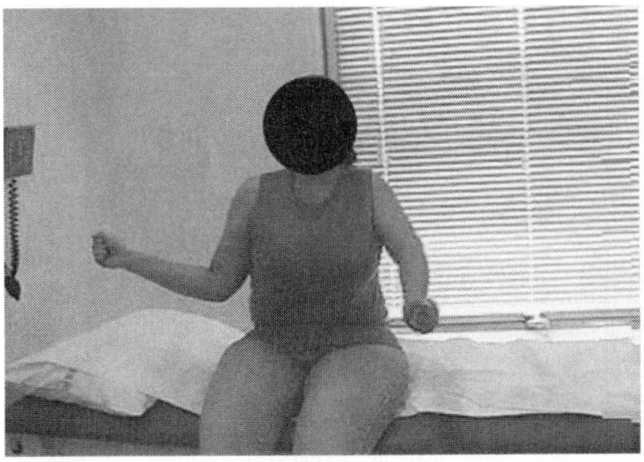

Fig. 3. A locked left shoulder posterior dislocation in a 25-year-old woman. She has been asked to externally rotate both shoulders actively. Note the fixed internally rotated left shoulder (the patient abducts her shoulder in an attempt to gain rotation).

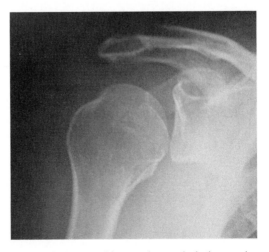

Fig. 4. A 36-year-old man has a locked posterior dislocation. Note the fixed internally rotated position (the "light bulb sign") in this true anteroposterior view.

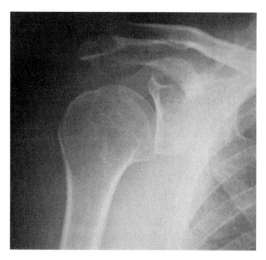

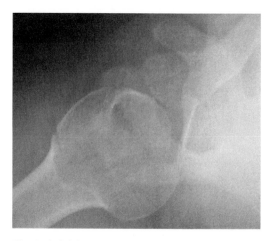

Fig. 7. Axial CT demonstrating a posterior dislocation in a patient who was given the diagnosis of "frozen shoulder" based on an incomplete radiographic series.

Fig. 5. In this true anteroposterior (AP) view there is a lack of a normal glenohumeral relationship (neither a clear joint space nor the overlap seen on non–true AP views).

articular surface. If the patient cannot abduct sufficiently to obtain a true axillary radiograph, the evaluating physician should insist on a Velpeau axillary or West Point view [52]. One must keep in mind, however, that a true axillary radiograph requires minimal abduction to obtain an adequate image (Fig. 7).

Cross-sectional imaging, such as CT, is an indispensable tool in the evaluation and treatment

of patients who have posterior glenohumeral dislocation. If one cannot obtain an adequate axillary radiograph because of pain or physical limitations, axial images of the glenohumeral joint can be obtained with CT. Moreover, CT allows more precise evaluation of the size of the characteristic impression defect and of the amount of remaining intact articular surface (Fig. 8) [53]. In addition, the presence of any associated fracture fragments can be evaluated more carefully, and

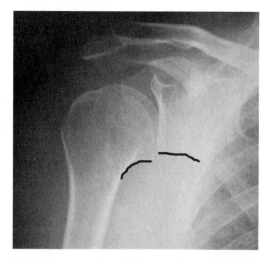

Fig. 6. Demonstration of Moloney's line, the equivalent of Shenton's line in the hip. Notice the break in continuity of the arc from the proximal humeral medial calcar to the inferior glenoid/scapula.

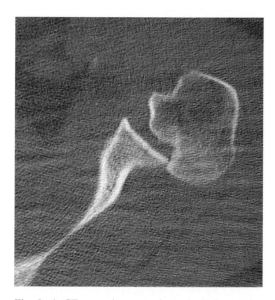

Fig. 8. A CT scan demonstrating a locked posterior dislocation and assessment of articular surface impression defect.

the characteristics of a posterior glenohumeral fracture-dislocation can be defined accurately (Fig. 9). Also, with CT, three-dimensional images can be generated, allowing the orthopedic surgeon to conceptualize completely the pathologic anatomy associated with posterior dislocation and thus to develop the best treatment strategy [54]. MRI has the added advantage of demonstrating concomitant soft tissue lesions associated with posterior glenohumeral dislocation. MRI will reveal the characteristic lesions of the posterior capsulolabral complex and of the rotator cuff [46]. MRI can elucidate the cause of an irreducible posterior dislocation, such as a torn rotator cuff, interposed glenohumeral capsule, or the tendon of the long head of biceps [55].

Treatment

Definitive treatment guidelines do not yet exist for these complex and heterogeneous injuries, primarily because of the lack of high-level evidence on which to base these guidelines. Most of the literature addressing the treatment of traumatic posterior glenohumeral dislocation consists of small case series and retrospective reviews. Some consensus, however, has been reached regarding the factors that serve a critical role in the determination of the optimal treatment

strategy: the duration of dislocation, the size of the humeral head impression defect, the presence of fracture, and the vascularity to the humeral head articular surface.

Of course, in addition to the details of the injury, factors related to the patient's health and functional status are critical in determining the optimal management for this condition. Although most patients are excellent candidates for orthopedic intervention, others may be better served with "skillful neglect" [16]. Notably, elderly patients, particularly debilitated patients who have limited functional status, should be approached with caution. In some instances of persistent dislocation, these patients may experience mild or tolerable pain and may demonstrate a range of motion that, although significantly limited, provides the ability to perform most activities of daily living. In addition, these patients may have comorbidities that preclude extensive operative intervention. Other patients may have behavioral or psychiatric comorbidity that may jeopardize the potential success of any operative intervention and of the requisite rehabilitation protocol. Therefore, in this subset of patients, nonoperative management may be the more appropriate approach to the posterior glenohumeral dislocation. Most other patients who have this injury will benefit from orthopedic surgical intervention.

Closed versus open reduction

Closed reduction is acceptable for acute posterior glenohumeral dislocations that have been present for less than 6 weeks. This mode of treatment is most suitable for dislocations with a humeral head impression defect that affects less than 20% to 25% of the humeral head articular surface. Dislocations with larger defects will demonstrate persistent instability after reduction and thus will require additional operative intervention to restore stability.

Closed reduction typically requires pharmacologic relaxation and analgesia. The reduction maneuver requires that the humeral head first be disimpacted from the glenoid rim. Overzealous reduction maneuvers without first liberating the humeral head may lead to propagation of the impression defect to an anatomic neck fracture or to the displacement of fracture lines already present in the surgical neck or tuberosities [19]. Initial gentle internal rotation and lateral traction should disimpact the humeral head. Mimura and

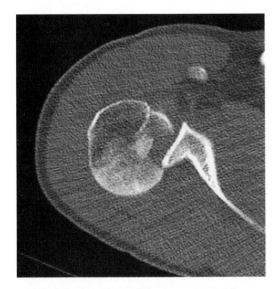

Fig. 9. A 36-year-old man following a posterior fracture dislocation. Axial CT demonstrates a locked posterior dislocation with a lesser tuberosity fracture (two-part lesser tuberosity fracture-dislocation).

colleagues [56] describe using a "lever principle" to unlock the humeral head. The technique consists of traction and medial pressure applied to the proximal upper extremity, which serves to adduct the proximal humerus, thus unlocking it from the posterior glenoid rim. Subsequent deliberate external rotation should lead to glenohumeral joint reduction. An alternative technique proposed by Hawkins and colleagues [12] consists of flexion and internal rotation of the injured extremity, followed by direct traction and manual pressure applied to the posterior aspect of the shoulder. Using this technique, however, they reported success in only 3 of 12 acute posterior dislocations.

Once successful reduction has been confirmed with postreduction radiographs, the shoulder should be immobilized in neutral to external rotation for 4 to 6 weeks [57]. This position allows apposition of the avulsed posterior capsulolabral complex with its origin, which typically heals reliably without the need for operative intervention [42,58]. Isometric external rotation strengthening can be performed within the brace. After the period of immobilization, the patient participates in a program of progressive range-of-motion exercises with subsequent internal and external rotation strengthening. Early series of closed reductions of posterior glenohumeral dislocation confirm favorable results with low rates of recurrence when the technique is applied appropriately to suitable candidates [1,12].

Open reduction of the humeral head should be performed in patients who have a persistent dislocation that has been present for more than 6 weeks, in whom the impression defect accounts for more than 20% to 25% of the humeral head, in whom concomitant fractures susceptible to iatrogenic displacement exist, or in whom closed reduction has been unsuccessful. A variety of surgical approaches has been advocated for open reduction of a posterior glenohumeral dislocation. The traditional deltopectoral approach provides excellent exposure to the anterior glenohumeral joint and is the authors' preferred approach when open reduction is required. Some have advocated an additional posterior approach to the joint or the superior deltoid-splitting approach as an alternative, because these approaches provide direct visualization of the entire glenoid and humeral head [59,60], although the authors have not found this visualization necessary. Following the approach to the glenohumeral joint, the humeral head must be disimpacted gently and reduced under direct visualization. Once reduced, the glenohumeral joint should be assessed for stability throughout a functional range of motion, and the need for additional reconstructive procedures should be determined. As an alternative to open reduction of the glenohumeral joint, some investigators have begun to explore arthroscopic reduction with favorable results [61,62].

Soft tissue repair

Although the posterior capsulolabral complex lesions typically heal with nonoperative management and thus rarely require surgical repair, repair is indicated in certain instances. If the patient's glenohumeral joint demonstrates persistent unacceptable instability following closed or open reduction, some advocate exclusive repair of the injured capsulolabral structures [59]. If more extensive intervention is required, however, mere repair of the glenohumeral capsulolabral complex is ill advised. Rather, soft tissue repair should be used as an adjunct to enhance postoperative stability. This soft tissue repair can be performed with a posteroinferior capsular shift through a posterior approach, including repair of the injured labrum, if present. Alternately, the arthroscopic approach to the repair of the capsulolabral complex has the added advantage of providing the ability to address the entire circumference of the glenohumeral capsulolabral architecture as well as concomitant glenohumeral pathology such as the rotator cuff.

Subscapularis transfer

In 1955, McLaughlin [3] described his technique for addressing posterior glenohumeral dislocation associated with a large impression defect of the humeral head. In this technique the subscapularis tendon is detached and transferred into the defect itself, thus precluding engagement of the posterior glenoid rim and subsequent instability. Hughes and Neer's [63] modification of this technique consists of the transfer of the osteotomized lesser tuberosity, rather than the subscapularis tendon alone, into the impression defect. This modified technique assures increased security of fixation and subsequent likelihood of successful healing [64–67].

Hawkins and colleagues [13] reported results of four patients treated with the original McLaughlin procedure and four treated with the modified procedure, all of whom demonstrated successful results, with range of motion of 160° to 165° of forward elevation, 40° to 45° of external rotation, and internal rotation to T12. They also reported five failures of the McLaughlin procedure performed at another institution in patients who had humeral head defects exceeding 45% of the humeral head or dislocations persistent for longer than 1 year. This report underscores the critical importance of appropriate indications for any procedure for posterior glenohumeral dislocation. Subscapularis or lesser tuberosity transfer should be reserved for patients who have a humeral head defect accounting for approximately 20% to 45% of the humeral head and in whom the dislocation has been present for less than 6 months to 1 year.

Transhumeral headplasty

Recently, disimpaction and elevation of the humeral head impression defect with bone grafting into the residual void has been described to restore the normal anatomic architecture to the articular surface [5,68,69]. Early results demonstrate excellent functional outcomes in small series. This technique offers a promising alternative to the detachment and transfer of the subscapularis or lesser tuberosity, thus avoiding the potential complications of restricted internal rotation range and strength. Its indications are limited, however. This technique should be reserved for acute dislocations that have occurred within 2 to 4 weeks and for patients who have an associated impression defect that accounts for less than 20% to 45% of the articular surface. Further contraindications to this procedure include elderly patients who have osteoporotic bone and patients who have a fractured or fragmented humeral head.

Humeral head reconstruction

Humeral head reconstruction with contoured allograft provides an alternative to subscapularis or lesser tuberosity transfer for patients who have a posterior glenohumeral dislocation of any duration with an associated impression defect representing between 20% and 45% of the humeral head articular surface. The acceptable size of the impression defect amenable to this technique may be expanded somewhat, particularly in young patients in whom one might be reluctant to perform a hemiarthroplasty. Several reports of this technique exist in the literature, describing the use of femoral head and humeral head allograft, as well as humeral head autograft from the contralateral extremity, all fixed with

countersunk or headless screws placed in the articular surface [70–74]. Gerber and colleagues [72] reported good to excellent results in three of four patients, with absent or mild pain in all patients, rivaling the results reported with subscapularis or tuberosity transfer cited by Hawkins and colleagues [13]. They discourage the use of this technique in the setting of severe osteopenia, because osteopenia may lead to collapse of the native humeral head, thus exposing the allograft to excessive load and resulting in ultimate failure of the allograft. Therefore, although no definitive guidelines exist for the use of this technique, intraoperative assessment of bone quality will aid the determination of its appropriateness.

Humeral osteotomy

Several reports in the literature describe various osteotomies that can be performed as an alternative to the previously mentioned procedures for posterior glenohumeral dislocation. One of these procedures is an external rotational osteotomy of the humerus that moves the impression defect of the anterior humeral head away from the posterior glenoid and thus prevents engagement with internal rotation [75–79]. Keppler and colleagues [76] reported on 10 patients who underwent rotational osteotomy of the humerus for a persistent posterior glenohumeral dislocation with an impression defect accounting for 20% to 40% of the humeral head. In six of these patients results were good or excellent, with no incidence of redislocation or necrosis of the humeral head. Patients who undergo this procedure experience significant limitation of external rotation. In another series of humeral rotational osteotomy for posterior instability, Surin and colleagues [78] demonstrated a loss of external rotation of at least 25% and as much as 100%. The authors do not consider humeral osteotomy to be a reasonable surgical option for these patients, and they do not perform this operation.

Glenoid reconstruction

The glenoid serves a critical role in maintaining glenohumeral stability. Some postulate that increased glenoid retroversion caused either by developmental dysplasia or by posttraumatic erosion of the posterior glenoid rim secondary to a persistent dislocation may render the glenohumeral joint susceptible to recurrent dislocation [80]. Glenoid osteotomy and bone graft attempts to restore appropriate version of the glenoid relative to the scapular axis, thus re-establishing the glenoid as a posterior buttress preventing dislocation. Significant complications have been reported in several series, however. Johnston and colleagues [81] reported on a series of 14 patients who underwent this procedure and underscored the importance of avoiding penetration of the glenoid articular surface to avoid iatrogenic post-traumatic arthritis. Wirth and colleagues [82] strongly discouraged the use of this procedure for recurrent posterior instability of the glenohumeral joint. Additional complications encountered by these authors included recurrent posterior instability, iatrogenic anterior instability, iatrogenic coracoid impingement syndrome, and avascular necrosis of the glenoid articular surface. Therefore this procedure is advocated only in rare cases of recurrent posterior glenohumeral dislocation in which the glenoid retroversion exceeds 30°. The authors have performed this procedure only sparingly and agree with others that it should be considered as a last-resort salvage procedure when most other options have failed.

Posterior bone-block reconstruction of the glenoid represents an alternative or adjunct to glenoid osteotomy to treat posterior glenohumeral dislocation (Fig. 10). Mowery and colleagues [83] reported on five patients who underwent posterior bone-block glenoid reconstruction for recurrent posterior glenohumeral dislocation, all of whom experienced good or excellent results. In light of these results, these authors advocate the use of this procedure in patients who have recurrent posterior dislocation and in whom previous operative intervention have failed and even in patients who have generalized ligamentous laxity or underlying connective tissue disease. Hernandez and Drez [84] increase the likelihood of success of this procedure by incorporating soft tissue reconstruction such as capsulorrhaphy and infraspinatus advancement.

Arthroplasty

Arthroplasty, either total shoulder or hemi-arthroplasty, is indicated for patients who have persistent posterior glenohumeral dislocation lasting longer than 6 months to 1 year with an impression defect that accounts for more than 45% of the articular surface of the humeral head [85,86]. Hawkins and colleagues [12] reported on nine patients who underwent hemiarthroplasty, six of whom demonstrated good results with absent or mild pain, 4+/5 strength in all manual muscle testing groups, and range of motion of 125° to 160° of forward elevation, 24° to 41° of external rotation, and internal rotation to L2. The three patients who experienced moderate pain later underwent total shoulder arthroplasty. Significant eburnation of the glenoid articular cartilage was noted, and all three patients experienced resolution of their pain postoperatively. For this reason, some advocate routine primary total shoulder arthroplasty for these patients to assure sustainable, reliable pain relief and anatomic restoration [87,88]. Six additional patients in Hawkins and colleagues' [12] study underwent primary total shoulder arthroplasty once it became available, with preoperative destruction of both the humeral head and glenoid. Although one patient experienced postoperative posterior dislocation, results were excellent in the other five patients. The authors attributed the dislocation to the placement of the humeral stem in 20° of retroversion. They recommend that for persistent dislocations lasting longer than 6 months, the humeral stem should be placed in neutral version, and in no case should retroversion exceed 20°. Further, they recommend posterior capsular plication as an adjunct for posterior stability.

Arthroplasty also may be indicated in the context of certain complex posterior glenohumeral fracture-dislocations [74,87,89]. Critical issues to consider in the decision to pursue arthroplasty for fracture-dislocation include the patient's age, comorbidities, and functional status, the displacement and vascularity of the fracture fragments, and the status of the humeral head articular surface. In younger patients, head salvage by way of open reduction and internal fixation typically is preferred. Certain three- and four-part fractures in elderly patients who have osteopenia and limited functional status may be an indication for arthroplasty instead.

Internal fixation

Once the decision has been made to proceed with a head-preserving procedure for posterior glenohumeral fracture-dislocation, one should follow a consistent four-step algorithm described by Robinson and colleagues [13] and others [60,90,91] to ensure optimum results. First, as noted previously, the open reduction can be performed using any of the available approaches. The humeral head should be freed from the posterior glenoid rim and reduced under direct vision

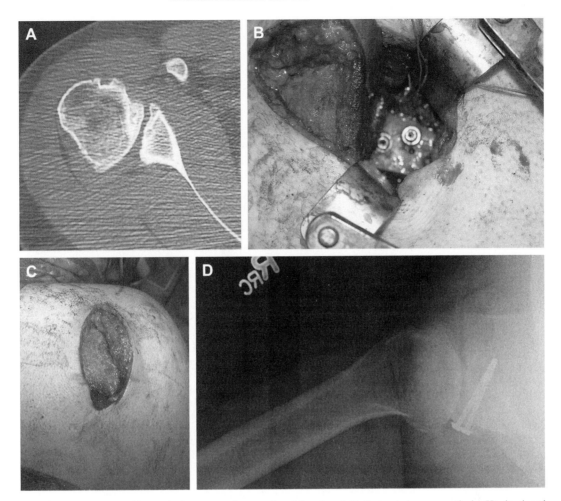

Fig. 10. (*A*) A 22-year-old man had a traumatic posterior dislocation initially treated nonoperatively. He developed recurrent posterior subluxation and underwent an arthroscopic posterior labral repair at an outside institution at age 19 years. At age 22 years, he had moderate to severe degenerative arthritis, posterior subluxation, and severe posterior glenoid erosion. (*B*) Intraoperative photograph of a posterior muscle-splitting approach demonstrating bone graft augmentation of the posterior glenoid fixated with two cannulated screws and washers. (*C*) Intraoperative photograph after retractors are removed from the muscle-splitting posterior approach. (*D*) Axial radiograph 3 years postoperative demonstrating maintenance of joint space. Patient now is pain-free, has no limitations of daily activities, and plays recreational sports.

by internal rotation of the head while carefully avoiding displacement of the fracture fragments. The vascularity of the humeral head then can be assessed to determine the appropriateness of head preservation. Second, provisional reduction and fixation of the fracture fragments then can be performed with Kirschner wires capitalizing on the posterior capsular and periosteal hinge. Third, the stability of the glenohumeral joint must be assessed to determine if any adjunctive procedure is necessary. Fourth, definitive fracture fixation is performed with the preferred implants,

including percutaneous pins, cancellous lag screws, and traditional or locking plates and screws (Fig. 11).

Robinson and colleagues [13] report impressive results with this regimented approach to open reduction and internal fixation of posterior glenohumeral fracture-dislocation. They demonstrated significant improvement in Disabilities of the Arm, Shoulder, and Hand and Constant scores with follow-up of 2 years. Short-Form 36 scores with respect to pain and function approached those for age- and sex-matched controls at 2 years.

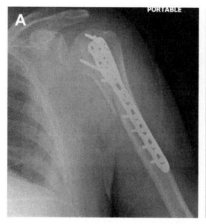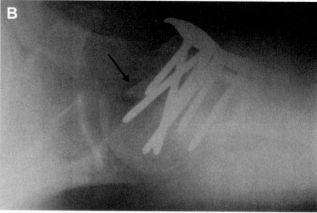

Fig. 11. (*A*) Anteroposterior and (*B*) axillary radiographs of a 35-year-old male police officer who suffered a locked posterior fracture–shaft dislocation 3 weeks before being referred for treatment. An open reduction of the locked posterior dislocation was performed, and a long proximal humeral locking plate was used for definitive fixation of the proximal humeral shaft fracture. Note the humeral head defect (15%–20%) on the postoperative axillary view.

These patients demonstrated average forward elevation of 172° and abduction of 169°. Twenty-two patients demonstrated full external rotation, and 16 demonstrated full internal rotation. These authors suggest that results following open reduction and internal fixation can be highly satisfactory provided the surgeon observes certain key principles: strict adherence to a regimented operative protocol, assurance of adequate vascularity of the fracture fragments with preservation of the posterior soft tissues and intertubercular groove, and judicious use of adjunctive procedures for stabilization.

Summary

Posterior glenohumeral dislocation is a complex and heterogeneous class of injury. The diagnosis of this rare condition continues to evade emergency physicians and orthopedic surgeons. To avoid this pitfall, one must approach patients with a high level of suspicion, diligent clinical evaluation, and a complete radiographic examination including anteroposterior, scapular lateral, and axillary images. With timely diagnosis, the treatment of this condition depends on the patient's health and functional status, the duration of injury, the size of the characteristic impression defect, the presence of concomitant fracture, and the vascularity of the fracture fragments. Myriad treatment alternatives exist, and the strategy chosen must address the patient's given pathology and ability to comply with the required rehabilitation protocol.

References

[1] Detenbeck LC. Posterior dislocations of the shoulder. J Trauma. 1972;12(3):183–92.

[2] Matsen FA III, Titelman RM, Lippitt SB, et al. Glenohumeral instability. In: Rockwood CA Jr, Matsen FA III, Wirth MA, et al, editors. The shoulder, vol. 2. 3rd edition. Philadelphia: Saunders; 2004. p. 655–794.

[3] McLaughlin H. Posterior dislocation of the shoulder. J Bone Joint Surg Am 1952;24(3):584–90.

[4] Rowe CR. Prognosis in dislocations of the shoulder. J Bone Joint Surg Am 1956;38(5):957–77.

[5] Robinson CM, Aderinto J. Posterior shoulder dislocations and fracture-dislocations. J Bone Joint Surg Am 2005;87(3):639–50.

[6] May VR Jr. Posterior dislocation of the shoulder: habitual, traumatic, and obstetrical. Orthop Clin North Am 1980;11(2):271–85.

[7] Hawkins RJ, Belle RM. Posterior instability of the shoulder. Instr Course Lect 1989;38:211–5.

[8] Heller KD, Forst J, Forst R, et al. Posterior dislocation of the shoulder: recommendations for a classification. Arch Orthop Trauma Surg 1994;113(4):228–31.

[9] Dorgan JA. Posterior dislocation of the shoulder. Am J Surg 1955;89(4):890–900.

[10] Samilson RL, Miller E. Posterior dislocations of the shoulder. Clin Orthop Relat Res 1964;32:69–86.

[11] Hawkins RJ. Unrecognized dislocations of the shoulder. Instr Course Lect 1985;34:258–63.

[12] Hawkins RJ, Neer CS II, Pianta RM, et al. Locked posterior dislocation of the shoulder. J Bone Joint Surg Am 1987;69(1):9–18.

[13] Robinson CM, Akhtar A, Mitchell M, et al. Complex posterior fracture-dislocation of the shoulder. Epidemiology, injury patterns, and results of operative treatment. J Bone Joint Surg Am 2007;89(7): 1454–66.

[14] Neer CS II. Displaced proximal humeral fractures. I. Classification and evaluation. J Bone Joint Surg Am 1970;52(6):1077–89.

[15] Neer CS II. Displaced proximal humeral fractures. II. Treatment of three-part and four-part displacement. J Bone Joint Surg Am 1970;52(6):1090–103.

[16] Loebenberg MI, Cuomo F. The treatment of chronic anterior and posterior dislocations of the glenohumeral joint and associated articular surface defects. Orthop Clin North Am 2000;31(1):23–34.

[17] Chattopadhyaya PK. Posterior fracture-dislocation of the shoulder. Report of a case. J Bone Joint Surg Br 1970;52(3):521–3.

[18] Galanakis IA, Kontakis GM, Steriopoulos KA. Posterior dislocation of the shoulder associated with fracture of the humeral anatomic neck. J Trauma 1997;42(6):1176–8.

[19] Hersche O, Gerber C. Iatrogenic displacement of fracture-dislocations of the shoulder. A report of seven cases. J Bone Joint Surg Br 1994;76(1):30–3.

[20] Ito H, Takayama A, Shirai Y. Posterior dislocation of the shoulder with a large fracture segment: a case report. J Shoulder Elbow Surg 2000;9(3):238–41.

[21] Richards RH, Clarke NM. Locked posterior fracture-dislocation of the shoulder. Injury 1989;20(5):297–300.

[22] Takase K, Watanabe A, Yamamoto K. Chronic posterior dislocation of the glenohumeral joint complicated by a fractured proximal humerus: a case report. J Orthop Surg (Hong Kong). 2006;14(2):204–7.

[23] Goodrich JA, Crosland E, Pye J. Acromion fracture associated with posterior shoulder dislocation. J Orthop Trauma. 1998;12(7):521–3.

[24] Kavanaugh JH. Posterior shoulder dislocation with ipsilateral humeral shaft fracture. A case report. Clin Orthop Relat Res. 1978;131:168–72.

[25] Moeller JC. Compound posterior dislocation of the glenohumeral joint. Case report. J Bone Joint Surg Am 1975;57(7):1006–7.

[26] Arden GP. Posterior dislocation of both shoulders; report of a case. J Bone Joint Surg Br 1956;38(2):558–63.

[27] Budd FW. Voluntary bilateral posterior dislocation of the shoulder joint. Report of a case. Clin Orthop Relat Res. 1969;63:181–3.

[28] Din KM, Meggitt BF. Bilateral four-part fractures with posterior dislocation of the shoulder. A case report. J Bone Joint Surg Br 1983;65(2):176–8.

[29] Iosifidis MI, Giannoulis I, Traios S, et al. Simultaneous bilateral posterior dislocation of the shoulder: diagnostic problems and management. A case report. Knee Surg Sports Traumatol Arthrosc 2006;14(8):766–70.

[30] Lindholm TS, Elmstedt E. Bilateral posterior dislocation of the shoulder combined with fracture of the proximal humerus. A case report. Acta Orthop Scand. 1980;51(3):485–8.

[31] Ozer H, Baltaci G, Selek H, et al. Opposite-direction bilateral fracture dislocation of the shoulders after an electric shock. Arch Orthop Trauma Surg 2005;125(7):499–502.

[32] Prillaman HA, Thompson RC Jr. Bilateral posterior fracture-dislocation of the shoulder. A case report. J Bone Joint Surg Am 1969;51(8):1627–30.

[33] Shaw JL. Bilateral posterior fracture-dislocation of the shoulder and other trauma caused by convulsive seizures. J Bone Joint Surg Am 1971;53(7):1437–40.

[34] Weissman SL, Torok G. Bilateral recurrent posterior dislocation of the shoulder: report of a case. J Bone Joint Surg Am 1958;40(2):479–82.

[35] Bhatia DN, de Beer JF, van Rooyen KS, du Toit DF. The reverse terrible triad of the shoulder: circumferential glenohumeral musculoligamentous disruption and neurologic injury associated with posterior shoulder dislocation. J Shoulder Elbow Surg 2007;16(3):e13–7.

[36] Roberts A, Wickstrom J. Prognosis of posterior dislocation of the shoulder. Acta Orthop Scand 1971;42(4):328–37.

[37] Finelli PF, Cardi JK. Seizure as a cause of fracture. Neurology 1989;39(6):858–60.

[38] Hepburn DA, Steel JM, Frier BM. Hypoglycemic convulsions cause serious musculoskeletal injuries in patients with IDDM. Diabetes Care 1989;12(1):32–4.

[39] Niazi TB, Lemon JG. Posterior dislocation of the shoulder due to a hypocalcaemic fit. Injury 1990;21(6):407.

[40] Tan AH. Missed posterior fracture-dislocation of the humeral head following an electrocution injury to the arm. Singapore Med J 2005;46(4):189–92.

[41] Norris TR, Green A. Proximal humerus fractures and glenohumeral dislocations. In: Browner BD, Levine AM, Jupiter JB, et al, editors. Skeletal trauma: basic science, management, and reconstruction. vol. 2. 3rd edition. Philadelphia: Saunders; 2003.

[42] Ovesen J, Sojbjerg JO. Posterior shoulder dislocation. Muscle and capsular lesions in cadaver experiments. Acta Orthop Scand 1986;57(6):535–6.

[43] Weber SC, Caspari RB. A biochemical evaluation of the restraints to posterior shoulder dislocation. Arthroscopy 1989;5(2):115–21.

[44] Simons P, Joekes E, Nelissen RG, et al. Posterior labrocapsular periosteal sleeve avulsion complicating locked posterior shoulder dislocation. Skeletal Radiol 1998;27(10):588–90.

[45] Schwartz E, Warren RF, O'Brien SJ, et al. Posterior shoulder instability. Orthop Clin North Am 1987;18(3):409–19.

[46] Hottya GA, Tirman PF, Bost FW, et al. Tear of the posterior shoulder stabilizers after posterior dislocation: MR imaging and MR arthrographic findings with arthroscopic correlation. AJR Am J Roentgenol 1998;171(3):763–8.

[47] Schoenfeld AJ, Lippitt SB. Rotator cuff tear associated with a posterior dislocation of the shoulder in a young adult: a case report and literature review. J Orthop Trauma 2007;21(2):150–2.

[48] Ogawa K, Ogawa Y, Yoshida A. Posterior fracture-dislocation of the shoulder with infraspinatus interposition: the buttonhole phenomenon. J Trauma 1997;43(4):688–91.

[49] Malgaigne JF. Traite des fractures et des luxations, vol. 2. Paris: JB Bailliere; 1855.

[50] Von Raebrox A, Campbell B, Ramesh R, et al. The association of subacromial dimples with recurrent posterior dislocation of the shoulder. J Shoulder Elbow Surg 2006;15(5):591–3.

[51] Hill NA, McLaughlin H. Locked posterior dislocation simulating a 'frozen shoulder'. J Trauma 1963; 3:225–34.

[52] Bloom MH, Obata WG. Diagnosis of posterior dislocation of the shoulder with use of Velpeau axillary and angle-up roentgenographic views. J Bone Joint Surg Am 1967;49(5):943–9.

[53] Wadlington VR, Hendrix RW, Rogers LF. Computed tomography of posterior fracture-dislocations of the shoulder: case reports. J Trauma 1992;32(1): 113–5.

[54] Kirtland S, Resnick D, Sartoris DJ, et al. Chronic unreduced dislocations of the glenohumeral joint: imaging strategy and pathologic correlation. J Trauma 1988;28(12):1622–31.

[55] Allard JC, Bancroft J. Irreducible posterior dislocation of the shoulder: MR and CT findings. J Comput Assist Tomogr 1991;15(4):694–6.

[56] Mimura T, Mori K, Matsusue Y, et al. Closed reduction for traumatic posterior dislocation of the shoulder using the 'lever principle': two case reports and a review of the literature. J Orthop Surg (Hong Kong) 2006;14(3):336–9.

[57] Cautilli RA, Joyce MF, Mackell JV Jr. Posterior dislocations of the shoulder: a method of postreduction management. Am J Sports Med 1978;6(6): 397–9.

[58] Scougall S. Posterior dislocation of the shoulder. J Bone Joint Surg Br 1957;39(4):726–32.

[59] Karachalios T, Bargiotas K, Papachristos A, et al. Reconstruction of a neglected posterior dislocation of the shoulder through a limited posterior deltoid-splitting approach. A case report. J Bone Joint Surg Am 2005;87(3):630–4.

[60] Stableforth PG, Sarangi PP. Posterior fracture-dislocation of the shoulder. A superior subacromial approach for open reduction. J Bone Joint Surg Br 1992;74(4):579–84.

[61] Varghese J, Thilak J, Mahajan CV. Arthroscopic treatment of acute traumatic posterior glenohumeral dislocation and anatomic neck fracture. Arthroscopy 2006;22(6):e671–2, 676.

[62] Verma NN, Sellards RA, Romeo AA. Arthroscopic reduction and repair of a locked posterior shoulder dislocation. Arthroscopy 2006;22(11): e1251–5, 1252.

[63] Hughes M, Neer CS II. Glenohumeral joint replacement and postoperative rehabilitation. Phys Ther 1975;55(8):850–8.

[64] Delcogliano A, Caporaso A, Chiossi S, et al. Surgical management of chronic, unreduced posterior dislocation of the shoulder. Knee Surg Sports Traumatol Arthrosc 2005;13(2):151–5.

[65] Finkelstein JA, Waddell JP, O'Driscoll SW, et al. Acute posterior fracture dislocations of the shoulder treated with the Neer modification of the McLaughlin procedure. J Orthop Trauma 1995;9(3):190–3.

[66] Nicola FG, Ellman H, Eckardt J, et al. Bilateral posterior fracture-dislocation of the shoulder treated with a modification of the McLaughlin procedure. A case report. J Bone Joint Surg Am 1981;63(7): 1175–7.

[67] Spencer EE Jr, Brems JJ. A simple technique for management of locked posterior shoulder dislocations: report of two cases. J Shoulder Elbow Surg 2005;14(6):650–2.

[68] Assom M, Castoldi F, Rossi R, et al. Humeral head impression fracture in acute posterior shoulder dislocation: new surgical technique. Knee Surg Sports Traumatol Arthrosc 2006;14(7):668–72.

[69] Re P, Gallo RA, Richmond JC. Transhumeral head plasty for large Hill-Sachs lesions. Arthroscopy 2006;22(7):e791–4, 798.

[70] Blasier RB, Burkus JK. Management of posterior fracture-dislocations of the shoulder. Clin Orthop Relat Res 1988;232:197–204.

[71] Connor PM, Boatright JR, D'Alessandro DF. Posterior fracture-dislocation of the shoulder: treatment with acute osteochondral grafting. J Shoulder Elbow Surg 1997;6(5):480–5.

[72] Gerber C, Lambert SM. Allograft reconstruction of segmental defects of the humeral head for the treatment of chronic locked posterior dislocation of the shoulder. J Bone Joint Surg Am 1996;78(3):376–82.

[73] Ivkovic A, Boric I, Cicak N. One-stage operation for locked bilateral posterior dislocation of the shoulder. J Bone Joint Surg Br 2007;89(6):825–8.

[74] Reckling FW. Posterior fracture-dislocation of the shoulder treated by a Neer hemiarthroplasty with a posterior surgical approach. Clin Orthop Relat Res 1986;207:133–7.

[75] Chaudhuri GK, Sengupta A, Saha AK. Rotation osteotomy of the shaft of the humerus for recurrent dislocation of the shoulder: anterior and posterior. Acta Orthop Scand 1974;45(2):193–8.

[76] Keppler P, Holz U, Thielemann FW, et al. Locked posterior dislocation of the shoulder: treatment using rotational osteotomy of the humerus. J Orthop Trauma 1994;8(4):286–92.

[77] Porteous MJ, Miller AJ. Humeral rotation osteotomy for chronic posterior dislocation of the shoulder. J Bone Joint Surg Br 1990;72(3):468–9.

[78] Surin V, Blader S, Markhede G, et al. Rotational osteotomy of the humerus for posterior instability of the shoulder. J Bone Joint Surg Am 1990;72(2):181–6.

[79] Vukov V. Posterior dislocation of the shoulder with a large anteromedial defect of the head of the humerus. A case report. Int Orthop 1985;9(1):37–40.

[80] Scott DJ Jr. Treatment of recurrent posterior dislocations of the shoulder by glenoplasty. Report of three cases. J Bone Joint Surg Am 1967;49(3): 471–6.

[81] Johnston GH, Hawkins RJ, Haddad R, et al. A complication of posterior glenoid osteotomy for recurrent posterior shoulder instability. Clin Orthop Relat Res 1984;187:147–9.

[82] Wirth MA, Seltzer DG, Rockwood CA Jr. Recurrent posterior glenohumeral dislocation associated with increased retroversion of the glenoid. A case report. Clin Orthop Relat Res 1994;308: 98–101.

[83] Mowery CA, Garfin SR, Booth RE, et al. Recurrent posterior dislocation of the shoulder: treatment using a bone block. J Bone Joint Surg Am 1985; 67(5):777–81.

[84] Hernandez A, Drez D. Operative treatment of posterior shoulder dislocations by posterior glenoidplasty, capsulorrhaphy, and infraspinatus advancement. Am J Sports Med 1986;14(3):187–91.

[85] Pritchett JW, Clark JM. Prosthetic replacement for chronic unreduced dislocations of the shoulder. Clin Orthop Relat Res 1987;216:89–93.

[86] Rowe CR, Zarins B. Chronic unreduced dislocations of the shoulder. J Bone Joint Surg Am 1982;64(4): 494–505.

[87] Cheng SL, Mackay MB, Richards RR. Treatment of locked posterior fracture-dislocations of the shoulder by total shoulder arthroplasty. J Shoulder Elbow Surg 1997;6(1):11–7.

[88] Checchia SL, Santos PD, Miyazaki AN. Surgical treatment of acute and chronic posterior fracture-dislocation of the shoulder. J Shoulder Elbow Surg 1998;7(1):53–65.

[89] Page AE, Meinhard BP, Schulz E, et al. Bilateral posterior fracture-dislocation of the shoulders: management by bilateral shoulder hemiarthroplasties. J Orthop Trauma 1995;9(6):526–9.

[90] De Wall M, Lervick G, Marsh JL. Posterior fracture-dislocation of the proximal humerus: treatment by closed reduction and limited fixation: a report of four cases. J Orthop Trauma 2005;19(1):48–51.

[91] Kaar TK, Wirth MA, Rockwood CA Jr. Missed posterior fracture-dislocation of the humeral head. A case report with a fifteen-year follow-up after delayed open reduction and internal fixation. J Bone Joint Surg Am 1999;81(5):708–10.

ELSEVIER
SAUNDERS

Orthop Clin N Am 39 (2008) 535–545

ORTHOPEDIC
CLINICS
OF NORTH AMERICA

Acromioclavicular and Sternoclavicular Joint Injuries

Peter B. MacDonald, MD, FRCSC[a],*, Pierre Lapointe, MD, FRCSC[b]

[a]Section of Orthopaedic Surgery, PanAm Clinic, University of Manitoba, 75 Poseidon Bay,
Winnipeg, Manitoba, R3M 3E4, Canada
[b]PanAm Clinic, University of Manitoba, 75 Poseidon Bay, Winnipeg, Manitoba, R3M 3E4, Canada

Acromioclavicular joint dislocation

Acromioclavicular (AC) joint injuries are a frequent diagnosis following an acute shoulder injury. Approximately 9% of shoulder girdle injuries involve damage to the AC joint [1]. These injuries occur commonly in active young adults in their second through fourth decades of life. Most often, the patient recalls a fall directly onto the top of the shoulder (acromion) with the arm adducted. This fall is the common mechanism for an AC joint injury, with another mechanism being a direct blow on the shoulder.

Anatomy

The AC joint is a diarthrodial articulation with a fibrocartilaginous meniscal disk that separates the articular surfaces of the acromial process and the distal clavicle. The capsule surrounding the joint is reinforced by the AC ligaments. These include the superior, inferior, anterior, and posterior ligaments. The superior and inferior ligaments are stronger than the anterior and posterior ligaments. The AC ligaments are the principle restraint to anteroposterior translation between the clavicle and the acromion [2,3]. Vertical stability of the clavicle is provided by the coracoclavicular (CC) ligaments, which are composed of the conoid and trapezoid. The AC and CC ligaments are the static stabilizers of the AC joint. The dynamic stabilizers are the deltoid and trapezius muscles. After an injury, the degree of clavicular displacement depends on the severity of injury to the ligaments and the muscles that attach to the clavicle.

Classification

Based on the degree of displacement, Allman [4] and Tossy and colleagues [5] initially divided these injuries into three types. Rockwood and Green [6] expanded the original classification to six types [7]. Type I represents a minor sprain of AC ligaments. Type II is a rupture of AC ligaments with sprain of CC ligaments. If both the AC and the CC ligaments are ruptured, this results in a type III AC joint injury. Types IV, V, and VI have the same ligamentous injuries as type III with more displacement of the clavicle and are also associated with detachment of deltoid and trapezius. In type IV injuries, the clavicle is displaced posteriorly into the trapezius muscle. The clavicle is elevated between 100% and 300% in type V injuries (Fig. 1). Type VI injuries are rare and the clavicle is displaced inferiorly behind the coracoid process and conjoint tendon (short biceps head and coracobrachialis tendon). This classification scheme is useful in the decision-making process for the treatment of AC joint injuries.

Assessment

Patients commonly complain of shoulder pain. The history and the mechanism of injury are important. Usually the pain is acute with a history of a recent fall or trauma to the shoulder. The pain is localized to the anterosuperior part of the shoulder around the AC joint.

Physical examination consists of inspection of both shoulders, which may highlight deformities that assist with diagnosis. In types I or II, swelling and bruising can be visualized and in other types a prominent clavicle is generally obvious. Sometimes an abrasion over the superior aspect of the shoulder can be seen secondary to the fall. The

---

* Corresponding author.
E-mail address: pmacdonald@panamclinic.com (P.B. MacDonald).

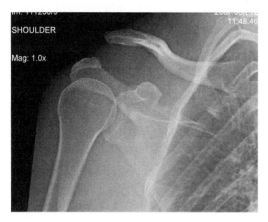

Fig. 1. Type V superior dislocation of the acromioclavicular joint.

AC joint is tender and the distal clavicle is
generally prominent. With high-grade AC separations superior and inferior translation can be
detected (positive piano key sign). The active and
passive range of motion should be evaluated. The
adduction and cross-body adduction test is usually painful around the AC joint. An injection of
a local anesthetic agent normally relieves the pain.
A neurovascular evaluation is always important
although neurovascular injury is rare in AC joint
injuries.

Radiography

The imaging begins with standard radiographs
(anteroposterior [AP], lateral, and axillary views).
Contralateral AP views allow determination of
the degree of clavicular displacement. The AP
view identifies the amount of vertical migration of
the clavicle, whereas the axillary view identifies
anterior or posterior displacement of the distal
clavicle. The Zanca view provides improved
imaging of the AC joint because it removes the
scapula from the field. In a trauma view the
radiographic beam is cephalic tilted about 10 to
15 degrees. Bilateral anteroposterior stress radiographs of the shoulders with 10 to 15 lb weights in
each hand are of limited usefulness, painful, and
not recommended in acute injury [8,9]. Our current recommendation for routine assessment of
the AC joint radiographically is an AP or Zanca
view, a lateral view, and an axillary view.

In type I injuries, the radiographic examination is normal. In type II, the clavicle is partially
elevated on radiographs but if the clavicle is
completely elevated (as much as 100%) this is

a type III injury. The axial view is important to
differentiate a type III from a type IV. In the axial
view of a type IV AC joint injury, the clavicle is
displaced posteriorly. The radiographs of a type
III and a type V are similar except that clavicular
elevation is more pronounced in type V injuries.
Usually in type V, the acromion to clavicle
displacement on the AP view is between 100%
and 300%. On the rare type VI, (three cases were
reported by Gerber and Rockwood Ref. [10]) the
clavicle is displaced inferiorly subacromial or
subcoracoid.

CT is the best test to evaluate the bony
structure of the AC joint. It assists with imaging
of distal clavicle fractures, displacement of the
clavicle, and any arthritic changes. MRI is also an
excellent imaging study to visualize the details of
the injury, including the ligamentous tears. In
acute AC joint dislocations, however, the routine
use of CT and MRI are not necessary.

Treatment

The literature on AC joint dislocation is extensive, reflecting the intense debate surrounding the
topic. A review of the history of treatment reveals
the controversy and the evolution of surgical
technique. The general goals of treatment of
patients who have AC joint injury are a normal
pain-free range of motion of the shoulder, return of
strength, and no limitations in activities [1]. The
choice of treatment is influenced by factors including the type of injury, the patient's occupation, the
patient's past medical history, the acuity of the
injury, and patient expectations [11]. The type of
injury is an important determinant of nonoperative
versus operative treatment. The final decision making should take into account the whole patient.

Type I and II injuries

Type I and II AC joint injuries are treated
nonoperatively [1,11–13]. In these types of
injuries, the joint retains some of its stability
[2,3]. Analgesic medication and nonsteroidal
anti-inflammatory drugs are used to relieve pain.
Cryotherapy can be applied on the shoulder to
reduce swelling and pain. A sling is worn for comfort. As the pain and swelling subside, early active
and passive motion and physiotherapy are recommended. Gladstone and colleagues [14] described
a four-phase rehabilitation program: phase 1,
pain control and immediate protected range of
motion and isometric exercises; phase 2,

strengthening exercises using isotonic contractions and proprioceptive neuromuscular facilitation exercises; phase 3, unrestricted functional participation with the goal of increasing strength, power, endurance, and neuromuscular control; and phase 4, return to activity with sport-specific functional drills. Most patients are able to return to normal activity in 2 to 4 weeks. An athlete is ready to return to competitive sports once the following criteria are met: full range of motion, no pain or tenderness, satisfactory clinical examination, and demonstration of adequate strength on isokinetic testing [14]. Most athletes are able to return to play in 2 to 4 weeks but other authors reported that some require up to 12 weeks [11].

Type III injuries

The treatment of type III AC joint injury is still somewhat controversial. This injury involves a complete tear of the AC ligaments and CC ligaments. In the Rookwood classification, based on progressive severity of ligament involvement, type III injuries are the turning point between the stable type I and II injuries and the unstable type IV, V, and VI injuries.

Schlegel and colleagues [15] prospectively studied the natural history of untreated acute grade III AC joint dislocation. At 1-year follow-up, the objective examination and strength testing of the 20 patients revealed no limitation of shoulder motion in the injured extremity and no difference between sides in rotational shoulder muscle strength. Tibone and colleagues [16] evaluated 20 patients with an average follow-up of 4.5 years after injury. This study shows that the strength of the shoulder is not significantly affected by conservative treatment. Phillips and colleagues [17] published a literature review and a meta-analysis of AC joint injury. They concluded that the literature does not support recommending an operative procedure to a patient who has an acute type III AC joint injury. Taft and colleagues [13] also concluded that most patients should be treated nonoperatively. A comparative analysis of operative versus nonoperative treatment by Galpin and colleagues [18] showed that nonoperative treatment provided an equal if not superior result with an earlier return to activities, sports, and work. Several other studies and review articles advocate conservative treatment over operative repair [1,11,12,19–21]. Two prospective randomized controlled studies between conservative and surgical treatment of acromioclavicular dislocation are published in the orthopaedic literature [22,23]. Bannister and colleagues [23] concluded that nonoperative management of AC dislocation is superior to early open reduction and coracoclavicular screw fixation. They suggest, however, that younger patients who have severe displacement are more likely to achieve an excellent result if the injury is stabilized early. Larsen and colleagues [22] recommended conservative treatment of most patients who had AC dislocation except for thin patients who had a prominent lateral end of the clavicle and those who did heavy labor.

Active young patients and overhead throwing athletes are sometimes considered as special cases. Some authors suggest that these patients who have AC joint complete dislocations should be considered for operative treatment [12,22–25]. Iannotti and Williams [12] have conducted an informal survey of physicians involved in the care of professional athletes and found that most favor a nonoperative approach. These physicians, however, would consider operative reduction for the throwing athlete. McFarland and colleagues [26,27] conducted a survey on the treatment of grade III AC separations in professional throwing athletes with the 42 team orthopaedists representing all 28 major league baseball teams. They found that 29 (69%) of the physicians would treat the injury nonoperatively, whereas 13 (31%) would operate early for a hypothetical starting rotation pitcher who had sustained this injury.

The nonoperative treatment of type III AC joint injury is similar to that for types I and II. Analgesic medication, nonsteroidal anti-inflammatory drugs, cryotherapy, and a sling for pain and patient comfort are used. As the pain and swelling diminish, early motion and exercises are initiated.

Type IV, V, and VI injuries

These injuries involve rupture of the AC ligaments, the CC ligaments, and deltotrapezius disruption with resultant severe displacement of the distal clavicle. In type IV, the posterior translation of the distal clavicle into the trapezius muscle creates pain and discomfort. Type V, with severe superior migration of the clavicle, can potentially lead to skin compromise. These rare type VI AC joint injuries generally require operative intervention [1,11,12,25,28,29].

Surgical management

Types IV, V, VI, some specific type III, and open AC joint injuries are indications for surgical treatment. The orthopedic literature is replete with a wide variety of surgical approaches to treat these injuries [1,12,22,23,30–38]. Many different surgical techniques have been described with one goal in mind: to stabilize the distal clavicle. Most surgical options can be grouped into a few general techniques [1,12,25,28]. Those involve primary fixation across the acromioclavicular joint, dynamic muscle transfer, fixation between the clavicle and the coracoid, and ligament reconstruction.

Primary fixation across the acromioclavicular joint

The AC joint dislocation can be stabilized by a transfixing device, including Kirschner wires, Steinmann pins, or screws (threaded preferred). These techniques can be done percutaneously or open. In association with the open methods, primary repair of the AC ligaments, coracoclavicular ligaments, or deltotrapezius fascia may be done. Some concerns and complications are associated with this technique. These include a second procedure for hardware removal, risk for hardware migration and breakage [39,40], and an increased incidence of AC joint arthritis.

The hook plate, a newer fixation device, is designed for primary fixation across the AC joint (Fig. 2) [12,25,28,41,42]. The construct involves plate fixation of the distal clavicle with a hook component that slides under the acromion for trans-AC joint fixation. Some authors find this technique demanding and associated with a higher rate of wound infections and healing problems [12,41,42]. Most all patients require hardware removal as the hook component may erode into the acromion over time. This plate may also be used for distal clavicle fractures [43,44].

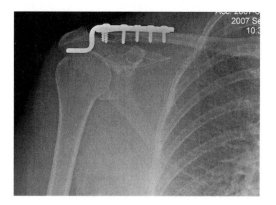

Fig. 2. Hook plate fixation of a type V acromioclavicular joint dislocation.

Fixation between the clavicle and the coracoid

Extra-articular stabilization, with a fixation between the clavicle and the coracoid, is another surgical method to address AC joint injuries. Several different techniques have been described for coracoclavicular fixation. In 1941, Bosworth [45] published a method of screw fixation. Several modifications of this original technique exist (Fig. 3). The surgery consists of an open reduction of the AC joint dislocation with the insertion of a screw from the distal clavicle to the coracoid process. A concurrent repair of the coracoclavicular ligaments and deltotrapezius fascia may be done. Because of the high rate of hardware migration and screw breakage over time, a second surgery is usually recommended between 8 and 12 weeks postoperatively [12,28]. At times, heterotopic ossification can be seen on follow-up radiographs between the clavicle and the coracoid process, but this complication does not have a significant clinical impact [46,47]. The placement of the screw may be done percutaneously; however, this increases the technical difficulty of the procedure and has been associated with a higher complication rate [48]. Using the coracoclavicular fixation principle, several other techniques have been described to replace the screw. These include metallic cerclage fixation, Dacron graft, sutures, suture anchors, or bioabsorbable implants [49–53]. Complications associated with these techniques are implant specific: failure, erosion of the bone, infection, and neurovascular injury that can occur during the passage of the loop around the coracoid process. Specific to the cerclage technique, the distal clavicle may translate anteriorly relative to the acromion because of anterior placement of the cerclage device on the coracoid. To avoid this problem, it is recommended that the cerclage loops be placed around the base of the coracoid process, as posterior as possible [25,50].

Dynamic muscle transfer

Most surgical stabilizations for complete AC joint dislocation are static procedures. Dynamic forms of stabilization have also been described by different authors [12,28,54,55]. The tendon of the coracobrachialis and the short head of the biceps are normally attached to the coracoid process. The surgical technique involves an osteotomy of the tip of the coracoid process, which is transferred to the undersurface of the clavicle. The inferior pull of the conjoint tendon on the clavicle should dynamically hold the AC joint reduced.

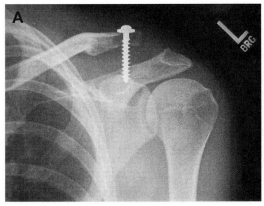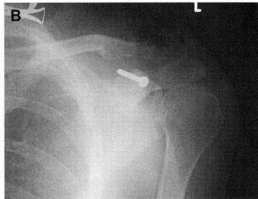

Fig. 3. Coracoclavicular screw fixation and distal clavicle excision to stabilize the distal clavicle (*A*). Because the screw had limited purchase in the coracoid, failure occurred (*B*).

Complications associated with this technique include traction injury to the musculocutaneous nerve, delayed union, nonunion, and excessive motion at the AC joint because of the dynamic nature of the reconstruction.

Ligament transfers and soft tissue reconstruction

Another static form of surgical stabilization of the AC joint consists of a ligament transfer or soft tissue reconstruction. The most common is the Weaver-Dunn technique, described in 1972 for acute and chronic AC joint dislocation [38]. This procedure consists of excision of the distal clavicle, release of the coracoacromial ligament from its acromial attachment, and transfer to the distal clavicle. Since its first description, many variations of the procedure have been published. Those variations include release of the coracoacromial ligament with or without a small flake of acromial bone and augmentation with coracoclavicular fixation. In 2007, Jiang and colleagues [31] described another type of dynamic transfer of the conjoint tendon. The surgical procedure consists of transfer of the lateral half of the conjoined tendon to the distal aspect of the clavicle with additional coracoclavicular fixation (double-loaded number 2 Ethibond suture anchor). They found this technique useful because it spares the coracoacromial ligament, which serves as a static stabilizer against anterosuperior migration of the humeral head. This technique can also be helpful in cases of a weak or thin coracoacromial ligament and in revision cases in which the coracoacromial ligament has already been harvested.

Anatomic reconstruction

Most recently, authors have advocated anatomic reconstruction of the different ligament complexes (coracoclavicular and acromioclavicular ligaments) using free grafts [1,12,34]. Recent biomechanical studies have demonstrated that anatomic reconstruction with free graft provided better stability than other ligament transfers [56–58]. Mazzocca and colleagues [56] did a controlled laboratory study to compare a newly developed anatomic coracoclavicular ligament reconstruction with a modified Weaver-Dunn procedure. They concluded that the anatomic coracoclavicular reconstruction has less anterior and posterior translation and more closely approximates the intact state, restoring function of the acromioclavicular and coracoclavicular ligaments. Costic and colleagues [57] published a controlled laboratory study to evaluate the cyclic behavior and structural properties of an anatomic tendon reconstruction of the coracoclavicular ligament complex. They concluded that the anatomic reconstruction approximates more closely the stiffness of the coracoclavicular ligament complex than current nonanatomic reconstructions.

Author's preferred method

The senior author has previously described his recommended technique for acromioclavicular dislocation [34]. This technique consists of an open distal clavicle resection and anatomic stabilization with a free semitendinosus allograft combined with heavy nonabsorbable suture as an augmentation and coracoacromial ligament transfer (acromion based) to augment the reconstruction of the AC ligaments.

Preferred technique

The patient is placed in a modified beach chair position with the head of the bed elevated 20 degrees and a 1-L intravenous bag under the affected scapula. A free limb drape is used with adequate exposure of the AC joint area. An incision is made in Langer lines from the posterior extent of the distal clavicle anteriorly to the level of the coracoid. Dissection is carried down first to the distal clavicle. In type IV and V AC joint injures, the clavicle is herniated through the trapezius fascia and is irreducible without bony resection or soft tissue release. The distal 1 cm of the clavicle is resected with an oscillating saw in a line perpendicular to the shaft of the clavicle.

Further dissection is then carried down to the coracoid, which involves splitting the overlying deltoid muscle fibers. Subperiosteal dissection proceeds around the coracoid approximately 3 cm posterior from its tip, followed by passing a curved suture passing device around the coracoid at its base. At this point, a double number 1 monofilament suture is passed around the coracoid.

As the dissection is performed, the free semitendinosus graft is prepared by passing leading sutures (number 2 nonabsorbable) to secure either end. Two number 2 heavy nonabsorbable Fibrewire sutures (Arthrex, Naples, Flordia) are used as an augment to the semitendinosus graft. The graft is first passed around the coracoid using the single suture as a shuttle to pass the leading sutures. Subsequently, the augment is passed along the same path.

The distal clavicle is prepared next. In an attempt to replicate the natural anatomy, two holes are drilled through the clavicle at the origins of the conoid and the trapezoid ligaments (Fig. 4). This procedure is done by first passing a guidewire and then reaming to the appropriate diameter derived from the measured limbs of the semitendinosus graft along with one limb of the suture augment. The composite graft limbs are then passed through their respective holes in the clavicle to anatomically reconstruct the coracoclavicular ligaments.

To strengthen the reconstruction, the coracoacromial ligament is mobilized off its insertion on the coracoid so that it can rotate on its attachment on the acromion. The free end of the ligament is then sutured with number 2 nonabsorbable sutures to secure it through drill holes in the distal clavicle. These sutures are not tied until the suture braid is tied and the clavicle is reduced.

The clavicle is then reduced into position with respect to the coracoid and the distal clavicle. The braided suture limbs are then tied to secure the construct so that the knot is located inferiorly between the clavicle and the coracoid. This suture augment acts as an internal splint until tendongraft incorporation occurs biologically. The transferred coracoacromial ligament can now be tied securely to the distal clavicle. The semitendinosus tendon graft is passed and tied so that the knot in the tendon lies superior to the clavicle.

As a final step, any free excess ends of the tendon graft are folded over and sutured to the reconstructed AC ligaments (acromial-based coraco-acromial ligament). The deltoid and the deltotrapezius fascia are then closed to cover the augment suture knot and the top of the clavicle. A subcuticular suture completes wound closure.

Postoperatively, the patient is placed in a sling, and gentle pendulum exercises are started immediately. Active assisted exercises are delayed until after postoperative week 4. Active motion then follows at week 6, with resisted exercises started at week 8. Full return to contact sports or heavy labor typically occurs around weeks 14 to 16.

Sternoclavicular joint dislocation

Sternoclavicular (SC) joint dislocation is an uncommon injury. It is of two general types: anterior and posterior. The posterior dislocation is much less common than anterior dislocation. The SC dislocation may follow direct force to the clavicle or more commonly from an indirect force to the shoulder. The direction of the force on the shoulder usually determines the type of dislocation. When an anterolateral force compresses the clavicle toward the sternum and propels the shoulder backward, this produces an anterior dislocation of the SC joint. Also, a posterolateral compression on the shoulder moves it forward and the force directed toward the clavicle produces a posterior dislocation. In addition, many presupposed SC dislocations in patients younger than 25 years old are actually fractures through the physeal plate. The medial clavicular epiphysis may not close until this age. Those physeal injuries represent Salter-Harris type I or II fractures.

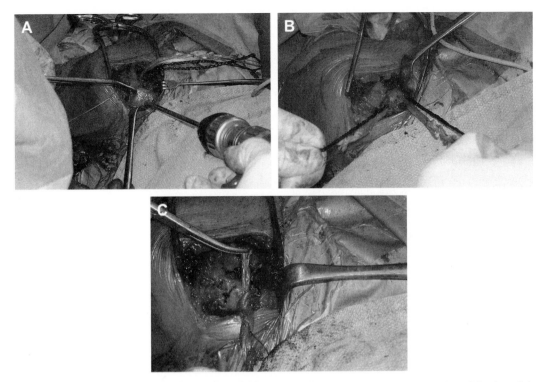

Fig. 4. Acromioclavicular joint reconstruction. Drill tunnels are created in the distal clavicle at the origin sites of the conoid and trapezoid ligaments (*A*). A semitendinosus tendon graft and an absorbable suture augment are passed around the base of the coronoid (*B*). The distal clavicle is reduced and the tendon graft and suture augment are tied (*C*).

The SC joint is the only bony articulation between the limb and the upper extremity. It is a saddle-type synovial joint. The capsule surrounding the joint is reinforced by different ligaments, including, superiorly, the interclavicular ligament, and inferiorly the costoclavicular ligaments and the anterior and posterior SC ligaments. The articular cartilage is mainly fibrocartilaginous. The articular surfaces are separated by a fibrocartilaginous articular disc. It is located inside the joint and divides it into two synovial cavities. This disc is an important shock absorber of forces transmitted along the clavicle.

Patients who have an SC joint injury commonly complain of anterior chest and shoulder pain after usually a violent injury. The most common cause of SC dislocation is motor vehicle collisions followed by athletic injuries and falls. The pain is exacerbated by arm movement or by assuming a supine position. Other symptoms, such as dyspnea, stridor, dysphagia, and paresthesias, may be the result of a posterior SC dislocation with compression of adjacent structures.

At physical examination, the affected shoulder usually appears shortened. In general, the patient has edema, tenderness, and ecchymoses over the SC joint. Pain is exacerbated with range of motion. Palpation can reveal an anterior and medial protrusion in anterior dislocations. In posterior dislocations, findings may be more subtle. It is important to check vital signs and the circulation to the upper extremity with posterior dislocations because mediastinal structures may be compressed. The patient should also be asked about shortness of breath from possible tracheal impingement.

Imaging studies are an important step in the evaluation of a patient who has an SC joint injury. Routine radiographs rule out other injuries, such as clavicle fractures, rib fractures, or a sternal fracture. Radiographs are difficult to interpret for SC joint dislocations because of overlying shadows. The serendipity view, a specialized view described by Rockwood, may help to determine the clavicle position. The beam is tilted to 40 degrees from vertical and directed cephalad through the manubrium of the patient while in a supine position. A CT scan, however, is a better imaging modality to evaluate SC joint injury. A CT scan allows evaluation of both SC joints, provides important information on the vital structures of the superior mediastinum, and helps to distinguish a physeal injury in younger patients.

Treatment of anterior sternoclavicular joint dislocation

The treatment of acute anterior SC joint dislocations is controversial. It is difficult to study with a well-designed prospective study because of the low frequency of this injury. A few studies in the literature can help us with the choice of treatment, however. Most anterior dislocations have little long-term functional impact [59,60]. One study reported long-term follow-up results in 10 patients treated nonoperatively [61]. The results of treatment were good in 7 patients, fair in 2 patients, and poor in 1 patient. They concluded that nonoperative management is the treatment of choice. Also, the contribution of the clavicle for most daily activities is minimal [59]. In most cases, the joint remains unstable regardless of the treatment [12,59,60]. A study by Savastano and Stutz [62] reported the results of 12 patients treated closed and open. They concluded that stability of the SC joint is not necessary to ensure normal function of the involved limb. They also found that residual prominence of the medial portion of the clavicle does not cause pain and does not interfere with shoulder function.

Despite the common residual instability of anterior dislocations, most authors recommend at least one closed reduction attempt [12,59,60]. A study by Nettles and Linscheid [63] treated 14 patients with closed reduction. Eleven had no recurrence or pain. The reduction may be performed with local anesthetic, under sedation, or under general anesthesia. The patient is placed supine with a thick pad between the shoulders. The reduction entails abduction of the shoulder to 90 degrees, 10 to 15 degrees of extension, and traction on the arm with posterior pressure over the medial end of the clavicle [60]. Immobilization after the closed reduction depends on the stability of the joint. If the anterior dislocation reduced and is stable, the patient is immobilized in a sling for 6 weeks. At week 3, the patient should start elbow exercises and glenohumeral rotation. In an unstable SC joint, a sling is used for a few weeks until symptoms resolve, followed by

a progressive program of range of motion and strengthening. Surgical stabilization of the clavicle is not recommended by most authors [12,59,60]. In most cases, the risks of surgery outweigh the potential benefits. The literature reports significant complications, such as hardware migration, infections, recurrence of the dislocation, and noncosmetic results. Operative treatment should be considered only in symptomatic patients who have failed conservative treatment. (See posterior dislocations section for more surgical details.)

Treatment of posterior sternoclavicular joint dislocation

Posterior dislocations are much less common than anterior dislocations. Posterior dislocations, however, are more serious and associated with significant complications and require prompt attention. Initially, a complete examination of the patient is important for the diagnosis of a posterior SC joint injury and for other associated lesions secondary to mediastinal compression by the clavicle. Behind the SC joint and the inner third of the clavicle are vital anatomic structures. Some of these vital structures include the innominate artery, innominate vein, vagus nerve, phrenic nerve, internal jugular vein, trachea, and esophagus. If other lesions are associated, appropriate consultants should be called in before any specific treatment. Most authors recommend that closed reduction is the initial treatment [12,59,60,64]. A cardiothoracic surgeon should be present during the reduction.

The closed reduction is performed under general anesthesia. Many different techniques have been described for closed reduction. The standard abduction traction technique is similar to the technique used for anterior dislocations. The patient is supine with the shoulder of the injury side near the edge of the table with a thick pad between the scapulas. Lateral traction is applied with the arm in abduction and extension. If reduction is not obtained, the clavicle can be grasped with the fingers to dislodge it from behind the sternum. If the clavicle is still dislocated, a towel clip is used to grasp it and it is lifted back into position. This procedure is always done with sterile technique. When the clavicle is reduced after a posterior dislocation, it is usually stable.

After reduction, the patient should be immobilized in a figure-of-8 strap for 6 weeks. Active assisted range-of-motion exercises are started at

3 to 4 weeks. Usually, full activities and sport can be allowed around 12 to 16 weeks.

Surgical treatment posterior sternoclavicular joint dislocation

The complication rate of posterior dislocations of the SC joint is high [65]. Also, most patients cannot tolerate posterior dislocation of the SC joint and the literature contains several reports of complications arising in unreduced cases. A failed closed reduction of a posterior SC joint dislocation is therefore an indication for open reduction. Because of the vital structures at risk, the surgery should be done with a thoracic surgeon on standby. The patient is positioned supine with a thick pad between the shoulders. The thorax, neck, and upper extremity should be prepped and draped for surgery. The upper extremity of the dislocated side should be drape-free for manipulation and traction. An anterior incision is created in a longitudinal fashion. The soft tissues are removed and the SC joint is explored. The SC joint is reduced by traction and countertraction. The final treatment depends on the stability of the joint postreduction. If the joint is stable, the same treatment protocol used for closed reduction is appropriate. If the joint is unstable, however, a reconstruction of the SC joint is recommended. There are various soft tissue procedures described in the literature for reconstruction. It is difficult to determine which is the best method. Spencer and Kuhn [66] reported a biomechanical analysis of reconstructions for SC joint instability. They concluded that the figure-of-8 semitendinosus reconstruction for SC joint instability has superior initial biomechanical properties.

Author's preferred method

For the rare cases that require reconstruction, we use the figure-of-8 semitendinosus reconstruction. The patient position and approach are similar as described previously for open reduction. Four drill holes are placed, two in the distal clavicle and two in the manubrium, in an anterior-to-posterior direction. The tendon is passed with a suture passer in a figure-of-8 fashion, which reconstructs the anterior and posterior ligaments of the SC joint. After surgery, the patient should be immobilized in a figure-of-8 strap for 6 weeks. Active assisted range-of-motion exercises are started at 6 weeks. Usually, active motion and progressive strengthening exercises can be allowed around 12 weeks.

References

[1] Mazzocca AD, Arciero RA, Bicos J. Evaluation and treatment of acromioclavicular joint injuries. Am J Sports Med 2007;35(2):316–29.

[2] Fukuda K, Craig EV, An KN, et al. Biomechanical study of the ligamentous system of the acromioclavicular joint. J Bone Joint Surg Am 1986;68(3): 434–40.

[3] Debski RE, Parsons IM IV, Woo SL, et al. Effect of capsular injury on acromioclavicular joint mechanics. J Bone Joint Surg Am 2001;83-A(9):1344–51.

[4] Allman FL. Fractures and ligamentous injuries of the clavicle and its articulation. J Bone Joint Surg 1967;49-A:774–84.

[5] Tossy JD, Mead NC, Sigmond HM. Acromioclavicular separations: useful and practical classification for treatment. Clin Orthop Relat Res 1963;28:111–9.

[6] Rockwood CA, Green DP. Fractures in adults. Philadelphia: Lippincott-Raven; 1984:860.

[7] Rockwood CA. Injuries to the acromioclavicular joint [Chapter 20]. In: Rockwood CA Jr, Williams GR, Young DC, editors. Rockwood & Green's fractures in adults. 4th edition. Philadelphia: Lippincott-Raven Publishers; 1996.

[8] Yap JJ, Curl LA, Kvitne RS, et al. The value of weighted views of the acromioclavicular joint: results of a survey. Am J Sports Med 1999;27(6): 806–9.

[9] Bossart PJ, Joyce SM, Manaster BJ, et al. Lack of efficacy of "weighted" radiographs in diagnosing acute acromioclavicular separation. Ann Emerg Med 1988;17(1):20–4.

[10] Gerber C, Rockwood CA. Subcoracoid dislocation of the lateral end of the clavicle. A report of three cases. J Bone Joint Surg Am 1987;69(6):924–7.

[11] Bradley JP, Elkousy H. Decision making: operative versus nonoperative treatment of acromioclavicular joint injuries. Clin Sports Med 2003;22(2):277–90.

[12] Iannotti J, Williams Jr G. Disorders of the shoulder: diagnosis and management. 2nd edition. Philadelphia: Lippincott Williams & Wilkins; 2007. p. 979–1006.

[13] Taft TN, Wilson FC, Oglesby JW. Dislocation of the acromioclavicular joint. An end-result study. J Bone Joint Surg Am 1987;69(7):1045–51.

[14] Gladstone J, Wilk K, Andrews J. Nonoperative treatment of acromioclavicular joint injuries. Oper Tech Sports Med 1997;5:78–87.

[15] Schlegel TF, Burks RT, Marcus RL, et al. A prospective evaluation of untreated acute grade III acromioclavicular separations. Am J Sports Med 2001;29(6):699–703.

[16] Tibone J, Sellers R, Tonino P. Strength testing after third-degree acromioclavicular dislocations. Am J Sports Med 1992;20(3):328–31.

[17] Phillips AM, Smart C, Groom AF. Acromioclavicular dislocation. Conservative or surgical therapy. Clin Orthop Relat Res 1998;353:10–7.

[18] Galpin RD, Hawkins RJ, Grainger RW. A comparative analysis of operative versus nonoperative treatment of grade III acromioclavicular separations. Clin Orthop Relat Res 1985;193:150–5.

[19] MacDonald P, Alexander M, Frejuk J, et al. Comprehensive functional analysis of shoulders following complete acromioclavicular separation. Am J Sports Med 1988;16(5):475–80.

[20] Prybyla D, Owens B. et al. Acromioclavicular joint separations. Available at: www.emedecine.com. Accessed May 2008.

[21] Imatani RJ, Hanlon JJ, Cady GW. Acute, complete acromioclavicular separation. J Bone Joint Surg Am 1975;57(3):328–32.

[22] Larsen E, Bjerg-Nielsen A, Christensen P. Conservative or surgical treatment of acromioclavicular dislocation. A prospective, controlled, randomized study. J Bone Joint Surg Am 1986;68(4):552–5.

[23] Bannister GC, Wallace WA, Stableforth PG, et al. The management of acute acromioclavicular dislocation. A randomised prospective controlled trial. J Bone Joint Surg Br 1989;71(5):848–50.

[24] Press J, Zuckerman JD, Gallagher M, et al. Treatment of grade III acromioclavicular separations. Operative versus nonoperative management. Bull Hosp Jt Dis 1997;56(2):77–83.

[25] Lemos MJ. The evaluation and treatment of the injured acromioclavicular joint in athletes. Am J Sports Med 1998;26(1):137–44.

[26] McFarland EG, Blivin SJ, Doehring CB, et al. Treatment of grade III acromioclavicular separations in professional throwing athletes: results of a survey. Am J Orthop 1997;26(11):771–4.

[27] Rawes ML, Dias JJ. Long-term results of conservative treatment for acromioclavicular dislocation. J Bone Joint Surg Br 1996;78(3):410–2.

[28] Kwon YW, Iannotti JP. Operative treatment of acromioclavicular joint injuries and results. Clin Sports Med 2003;22(2):291–300, vi.

[29] Horn JS. The traumatic anatomy and treatment of acute acromio-clavicular dislocation. J Bone Joint Surg Br 1954;36-B:194–201.

[30] Dumontier C, Sautet A, Man M, et al. Acromioclavicular dislocations: treatment by coracoacromial ligamentoplasty. J Shoulder Elbow Surg 1995;4(2):130–4.

[31] Jiang C, Wang M, Rong G. Proximally based conjoined tendon transfer for coracoclavicular reconstruction in the treatment of acromioclavicular dislocation. J Bone Joint Surg Am 2007;89(11):2408–12.

[32] McConnell AJ, Yoo DJ, Zdero R, et al. Methods of operative fixation of the acromio-clavicular joint: a biomechanical comparison. J Orthop Trauma 2007;21(4):248–53.

[33] De Baets T, Truijen J, Driesen R, et al. The treatment of acromioclavicular joint dislocation Tossy grade III with a clavicle hook plate. Acta Orthop Belg 2004;70(6):515–9.

[34] MacDonald PB. Advanced reconstruction shoulder. Chapter 25: AC joint reconstruction for type V injury: acute. 239–46.

[35] Jones HP, Lemos MJ, Schepsis AA. Salvage of failed acromioclavicular joint reconstruction using autogenous semitendinosus tendon from the knee. Surgical technique and case report. Am J Sports Med 2001;29(2):234–7.

[36] Nicholas SJ, Lee SJ, Mullaney MJ, et al. Clinical outcomes of coracoclavicular ligament reconstructions using tendon grafts. Am J Sports Med 2007;35(11):1912–7 [Epub 2007 Aug 8].

[37] Pennington WT, Hergan DJ, Bartz BA. Arthroscopic coracoclavicular ligament reconstruction using biologic and suture fixation. Arthroscopy 2007;23(7):785.e1–7 [Epub 2007 Feb 14].

[38] Weaver JK, Dunn HK. Treatment of acromioclavicular injuries, especially complete acromioclavicular separation. J Bone Joint Surg Am 1972;54(6):1187–94.

[39] Foster GT, Chetty KG, Mahutte K, et al. Hemoptysis due to migration of a fractured Kirschner wire. Chest 2001;119(4):1285–6.

[40] Regel JP, Pospiech J, Aalders TA, et al. Intraspinal migration of a Kirschner wire 3 months after clavicular fracture fixation. Neurosurg Rev 2002;25(1–2):110–2.

[41] Faraj AA, Ketzer B. The use of a hook-plate in the management of acromioclavicular injuries. Report of ten cases. Acta Orthop Belg 2001;67(5):448–51.

[42] Sim E, Schwarz N, Höcker K, et al. Repair of complete acromioclavicular separations using the acromioclavicular-hook plate. Clin Orthop Relat Res 1995;314:134–42.

[43] Muramatsu K, Shigetomi M, Matsunaga T, et al. Use of the AO hook-plate for treatment of unstable fractures of the distal clavicle. Arch Orthop Trauma Surg 2007;127(3):191–4 [Epub 2007 Jan 13].

[44] Haidar SG, Krishnan KM, Deshmukh SC. Hook plate fixation for type II fractures of the lateral end of the clavicle. J Shoulder Elbow Surg 2006;15(4):419–23.

[45] Bosworth BM. Acromioclavicular separation. A new method of repair. Surg Gynecol Obstet 1941;73:866–71.

[46] Weitzman G. Treatment of acute acromioclavicular joint dislocation by a modified Bosworth method: Report on twenty-four cases. J Bone Joint Surg Am 1967;49:1167–78.

[47] Kennedy JC, Cameron H. Complete dislocation of the acromioclavicular joint. J Bone Joint Surg Br 1954;36-B:202–8.

[48] Tsou PM. Percutaneous cannulated screw coracoclavicular fixation for acute acromioclavicular

dislocations. Clin Orthop Relat Res 1989;243: 112–21.

[49] Breslow MJ, Jazrawi LM, Bernstein AD, et al. Treatment of acromioclavicular joint separation: suture or suture anchors? J Shoulder Elbow Surg 2002; 11(3):225–9.

[50] Morrison DS, Lemos MJ. Acromioclavicular separation. Reconstruction using synthetic loop augmentation. Am J Sports Med 1995;23(1):105–10.

[51] Stam L, Dawson I. Complete acromioclavicular dislocations treatment with a Dacron ligament. Injury 1991;22(3):173–6.

[52] Kappakas GS, McMaster JH. Repair of acromioclavicular separation using a Dacron prosthesis graft. Clin Orthop Relat Res 1978;131:247–51.

[53] Motamedi AR, Blevins FT, Willis MC, et al. Biomechanics of the coracoclavicular ligament complex and augmentations used in its repair and reconstruction. Am J Sports Med 2000;28(3):380–4.

[54] Brunelli G, Brunelli F. The treatment of acromioclavicular dislocation by transfer of the short head of biceps. Int Orthop 1988;12(2):105–8.

[55] Berson BL, Gilbert MS, Green S. Acromioclavicular dislocations treatment by transfer of the conjoined tendon and distal end of the coracoid process to the clavicle. Clin Orthop Relat Res 1978;135:157–64.

[56] Mazzocca AD, Santangelo SA, Johnson ST, et al. A biomechanical evaluation of an anatomical coracoclavicular ligament reconstruction. Am J Sports Med 2006;34(2):236–46 [Epub 2005 Nov 10].

[57] Costic RS, Labriola JE, Rodosky MW, et al. Biomechanical rationale for development of anatomical reconstructions of coracoclavicular ligaments after complete acromioclavicular joint dislocations. Am J Sports Med 2004;32(8):1929–36.

[58] Grutter PW, Petersen SA. Anatomical acromioclavicular ligament reconstruction: a biomechanical comparison of reconstructive techniques of the acromioclavicular joint. Am J Sports Med 2005;33(11): 1723–8 [Epub 2005 Aug 10].

[59] Miller ME, Ada JR. Injuries to the shoulder girdle. Part I: fractures of the scapula, clavicle, and glenoid. In: Browner BD, Jupiter JB, Levine AM, et al. editors. 2nd edition. Skeletal trauma: fractures, dislocations, ligamentous injuries, vol. 2. Philadelphia: WB Saunders; 1992. p. 1667–9.

[60] Bicos J, Nicholson GP. Treatment and results of sternoclavicular joint injuries Review. Clin Sports Med 2003;22(2):359–70.

[61] de Jong KP, Sukul DM. Anterior sternoclavicular dislocation a long term follow-up study. J Orthop Trauma 1990;4(4):420–3.

[62] Savastano AA, Stutz SJ. Traumatic sternoclavicular dislocation. Int Surg 1978;63(1):10–3.

[63] Nettles JL, Linscheid RL. Sternoclavicular dislocations. J Trauma 1968;8(2):158–64.

[64] Buckerfield CT, Castle ME. Acute traumatic retrosternal dislocation of the clavicle. J Bone Joint Surg Am 1984;66(3):379–85.

[65] Lemos MJ, Tolo ET. Complications of the treatment of the acromioclavicular and sternoclavicular joint injuries, including instability. Clin Sports Med 2003;22(2):371–85.

[66] Spencer EE Jr, Kuhn JE. Biomechanical analysis of reconstructions for sternoclavicular joint instability. J Bone Joint Surg Am 2004;86-A(1):98–105.

ELSEVIER
SAUNDERS

Orthop Clin N Am 39 (2008) 547–552

ORTHOPEDIC
CLINICS
OF NORTH AMERICA

Index

Note: Page numbers of article titles are in **boldface** type.

United States Postal Service

Statement of Ownership, Management, and Circulation
(All Periodicals Publications Except Requestor Publications)

1. Publication Title	2. Publication Number	3. Filing Date
Orthopedic Clinics of North America	9 5 0 - 9 2 0	9/15/08

4. Issue Frequency	5. Number of Issues Published Annually	6. Annual Subscription Price
Jan, Apr, Jul, Oct	4	$226.00

7. Complete Mailing Address of Known Office of Publication (Not printer) (Street, city, county, state, and ZIP+4)

Elsevier Inc.
360 Park Avenue South
New York, NY 10010-1710

Contact Person
Stephen Bushing
Telephone (Include area code)
215-239-3688

8. Complete Mailing Address of Headquarters or General Business Office of Publisher (Not printer)

Elsevier Inc., 360 Park Avenue South, New York, NY 10010-1710

9. Full Names and Complete Mailing Addresses of Publisher, Editor, and Managing Editor (Do not leave blank)

Publisher (Name and complete mailing address)

John Schrefer, Elsevier, Inc., 1600 John F. Kennedy Blvd. Suite 1800, Philadelphia, PA 19103-2899

Editor (Name and complete mailing address)

Deb Dellapena, Elsevier, Inc., 1600 John F. Kennedy Blvd. Suite 1800, Philadelphia, PA 19103-2899

Managing Editor (Name and complete mailing address)

Catherine Bewick, Elsevier, Inc., 1600 John F. Kennedy Blvd. Suite 1800, Philadelphia, PA 19103-2899

10. Owner (Do not leave blank. If the publication is owned by a corporation, give the name and address of the corporation immediately followed by the names and addresses of all stockholders owning or holding 1 percent or more of the total amount of stock. If not owned by a corporation, give the names and addresses of the individual owners. If owned by a partnership or other unincorporated firm, give its name and address as well as those of each individual owner. If the publication is published by a nonprofit organization, give its name and address.)

Full Name	Complete Mailing Address
Wholly owned subsidiary of	4520 East-West Highway
Reed/Elsevier, US holdings	Bethesda, MD 20814

11. Known Bondholders, Mortgagees, and Other Security Holders Owning or Holding 1 Percent or More of Total Amount of Bonds, Mortgages, or Other Securities. If none, check box ☐ None

Full Name	Complete Mailing Address
N/A	

12. Tax Status (For completion by nonprofit organizations authorized to mail at nonprofit rates) (Check one)
The purpose, function, and nonprofit status of this organization and the exempt status for federal income tax purposes:
☐ Has Not Changed During Preceding 12 Months
☐ Has Changed During Preceding 12 Months (Publisher must submit explanation of change with this statement)

PS Form 3526, September 2006 (Page 1 of 3 (Instructions Page 3)) PSN 7530-01-000-9931 PRIVACY NOTICE: See our Privacy policy in www.usps.com

13. Publication Title	14. Issue Date for Circulation Data Below
Orthopedic Clinics of North America	July 2008

15. Extent and Nature of Circulation		Average No. Copies Each Issue During Preceding 12 Months	No. Copies of Single Issue Published Nearest to Filing Date
a. Total Number of Copies (Net press run)		3075	3000
b. Paid Circulation (By Mail and Outside the Mail)	(1) Mailed Outside-County Paid Subscriptions Stated on PS Form 3541. (Include paid distribution above nominal rate, advertiser's proof copies, and exchange copies)	1196	1105
	(2) Mailed In-County Paid Subscriptions Stated on PS Form 3541 (Include paid distribution above nominal rate, advertiser's proof copies, and exchange copies)		
	(3) Paid Distribution Outside the Mails Including Sales Through Dealers and Carriers, Street Vendors, Counter Sales, and Other Paid Distribution Outside USPS®	945	976
	(4) Paid Distribution by Other Classes Mailed Through the USPS (e.g. First-Class Mail®)		
c. Total Paid Distribution (Sum of 15b (1), (2), (3), and (4))	▶	2141	2081
d. Free or Nominal Rate Distribution (By Mail and Outside the Mail)	(1) Free or Nominal Rate Outside-County Copies Included on PS Form 3541	91	89
	(2) Free or Nominal Rate In-County Copies Included on PS Form 3541		
	(3) Free or Nominal Rate Copies Mailed at Other Classes Mailed Through the USPS (e.g. First-Class Mail)		
	(4) Free or Nominal Rate Distribution Outside the Mail (Carriers or other means)		
e. Total Free or Nominal Rate Distribution (Sum of 15d (1), (2), (3) and (4))	▶	91	89
f. Total Distribution (Sum of 15c and 15e)	▶	2232	2170
g. Copies not Distributed (See instructions to publishers #4 (page #3))	▶	843	830
h. Total (Sum of 15f and g)	▶	3075	3000
i. Percent Paid (15c divided by 15f times 100)		95.92%	95.90%

16. Publication of Statement of Ownership
☐ If the publication is a general publication, publication of this statement is required. Will be printed in the October 2008 issue of this publication.   ☐ Publication not required

17. Signature and Title of Editor, Publisher, Business Manager, or Owner   Date

[signature] Stephen Bushing – Executive Director of Subscription Services   September 15, 2008

I certify that all information furnished on this form is true and complete. I understand that anyone who furnishes false or misleading information on this form or who omits material or information requested on the form may be subject to criminal sanctions (including fines and imprisonment) and/or civil sanctions (including civil penalties).

PS Form 3526, September 2006 (Page 2 of 3)

Moving?

Make sure your subscription moves with you!

To notify us of your new address, find your **Clinics Account Number** (located on your mailing label above your name), and contact customer service at:

E-mail: elspcs@elsevier.com

800-654-2452 (subscribers in the U.S. & Canada)
1-407-563-6020 (subscribers outside of the U.S. & Canada)

Fax number: 407-363-9661

Elsevier Periodicals Customer Service
6277 Sea Harbor Drive
Orlando, FL 32887-4800

*To ensure uninterrupted delivery of your subscription, please notify us at least 4 weeks in advance of move.